# RCGP Insider's Guide
# to the CSA for the MRCGP

# RCGP Insider's Guide to the CSA for the MRCGP

Alexandra Rolfe

Sarah Atkins

Kamila Hawthorne

Celia Roberts

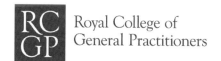

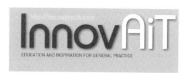

The Royal College of General Practitioners was founded in 1952 with this object:
*'To encourage, foster and maintain the highest possible standards in general practice and for that purpose to take or join with others in taking steps consistent with the charitable nature of that object which may assist towards the same.'*

Among its responsibilities under its Royal Charter the College is entitled to:
*'Diffuse information on all matters affecting general practice and issue such publications as may assist the object of the College.'*

*British Library Cataloguing-in-Publication Data*
A catalogue record for this book is available from the British Library

© Royal College of General Practitioners, 2015

Published by the Royal College of General Practitioners, 2015
30 Euston Square, London NW1 2FB

Designed and typeset by HWA Text and Data Management, London
Printed by Hobbs the Printers Ltd
Indexed by Susan Leech

ISBN 978-0-85084-389-7

To all the CSA candidates who so generously allowed us to record and analyse their consultations for our Knowledge Transfer Partnership research project with the RCGP led by King's College London and with Cardiff University.

# Contents

# About the authors

**Dr Alexandra Rolfe** MB ChB BSc (Hons) MRCGP DCH is a GP and clinical education fellow from Edinburgh. She completed her MRCGP in 2012 with a score of over 100 in the CSA. She works as a GP in Edinburgh and as a clinical education fellow at the University of Edinburgh. Her work includes improving prescribing in undergraduate students, medical education assessments and inter-professional education. She was also deputy editor of *InnovAiT*.

**Dr Sarah Atkins** BA(Hons) MA PhD is a post-doctoral research fellow at the University of Nottingham, within the Centre for Research in Applied Linguistics. Her research investigates language and professional communication, primarily in healthcare settings, with an emphasis on applying findings into practice.

**Prof. Kamila Hawthorne** MA (Oxon) MD FRCP FRCGP FAcadMEd DRCOG DCH (London) is an academic GP from Cardiff. She has been a GP for 26 years, and is a partner in an NHS practice in inner-city Cardiff and Associate Dean and Director for Community Learning at the School of Medicine, Cardiff University. Her research interests are in diabetes, health inequalities and medical education assessments. She has been an MRCGP examiner since 1997, and was involved in the design and delivery of the CSA from its inception in 2007. She is now Chair of the Assessment and Curriculum Development Committee of the RCGP and Vice Chair of the Specialty Advisory Committee of the RCGP.

**Prof. Celia Roberts** BA PGCert FAcSS is Professor Emerita in Sociolinguistics at King's College London. Her research is in the areas of language and communication in institutions with particular reference to multilingual societies. She was the Principal Investigator on the research project 'Performance features in clinical skills assessment' on which Chapters 4 and 5 are based.

# Foreword

Preparing for the Clinical Skills Assessment (CSA) can be a daunting prospect for ST3s and their trainers. The RCGP is committed to developing high-quality resources like the *RCGP Insider's Guide to the CSA for the MRCGP* to support candidates with their CSA preparation. This authoritative book is written by a group of 'CSA insiders' who are able to share their personal knowledge and experience of the CSA with candidates. This includes unique access to the findings of a sociolinguistic research project that has identified some features of candidate performance in the Data-Gathering and Interpersonal Skills domains of the CSA that are associated with examination success.

The authors provide insight into the development and structure of the CSA, and into the way that cases are designed and marked. They have developed two circuits of authentic CSA practice cases with input from the CSA Case Management Group. Their aim is to build confidence with practical preparation exercises and tips so that candidates approach the exam with the right mindset and succeed. I recommend this book to GP trainees and trainers, and to all those involved in the preparation of candidates for the CSA.

**Dr Pauline Foreman**
Chief Examiner, MRCGP

# Acknowledgements

Much of this book is based on the findings of linguistic research on the MRCGP Clinical Skills Assessment (CSA). The authors are grateful to various funding bodies who contributed to that research, including the Technology Strategy Board through the Knowledge Transfer Partnerships, the Academy of Medical Royal Colleges and the Economic and Social Research Council's 'Future Research Leaders' programme.

Many academic colleagues also helped shape the research and we would particularly like to thank Dr Spencer Hazel of Roskilde University for his contribution to the study. We're also grateful to Kay Mohanna from Keele University and Pauline Foreman, MRCGP Chief Examiner, who made the results from their own research on the MRCGP CSA available to us.

We are enormously grateful to the Royal College of General Practitioners for its support of this book, in particular to Dr Sue Rendel, Dr Adrian Freeman, Ruth Palmer, Fiona Erasmus and David Jeffrey. Special mention must also go to Dr Simon Ward for his invaluable and honest advice on the practice cases and their suitability for CSA preparation.

Finally, we would especially like to thank all the candidates and role-players who consented for us to use their exam footage in the project, whose transcripts appear here in this book, and those who tried out and gave us feedback on the ideas and cases featured in the book.

# Glossary

**abstracts** – the little summaries you provide at the outset of an explanation. We all have to read abstracts of papers. But we also do little summaries in conversation, and they can help signal that we are about to start a story so will be doing a lot of the talking. Often candidates use a 'mini-explanation' structure in their abstracts in order to indicate they were about to start a longer explanation, again where they would be doing a lot of the talking.

**alignment** – talking together with the patient, to the same purpose. This doesn't mean you have to agree wholeheartedly with the patient, although you might, but it does mean having a surface-level agreement about the particular task being carried out – such as asking questions and receiving answers during data-gathering, listening and showing understanding during a patient narrative.

**codas** – not just a conclusion to a story (or explanation), but a way of relating it back to the listener. We do these all the time when we tell conversational stories so that we can show why a story was relevant and bring the conversation back to the present: '… and that's how the camel got his humps'. Bringing an explanation back to the particular patient means demonstrating the relevance for him or her: '… which I understand is what your father suffered from'. This gives the patient an opportunity to then speak.

**information sandwiches** – this was a small-scale technique we saw a candidate use in the section on data-gathering for giving a chunk of information, followed by a 'checking prior understanding' question. You don't have to do it – it's not a secret to success – but it was one technique that she used well.

**making inferences** – working out how things are going, which might not be immediately obvious on the surface. Making inferences helps you to figure out what the patient is likely to want, how keen he or she sounds at certain points of the interaction and what a case is likely to be about. Of course, you can't always rely on inferences and sometimes you can guess wrongly, but it can still demonstrate that you're trying to be attentive to the patient (not to mention help you figure out where the case might be going!).

**metacommunication** – is a kind of 'talk about talk', or a commentary on how you want the things you are saying to be interpreted. 'It's a funny term, cystic fibrosis.' 'So that's maybe a few things to think about there.' This is the most complicated term we've borrowed from linguistics, but it was such a prominent feature of successful candidates' talk that we thought it was important to include. And you can see why it's useful – it gives the listener extra guidance on how to make sense of your talk.

**mini-explanations** – a structure lots of candidates use for giving definitions of medical terminology. It is a useful way of providing an 'abstract' or start to a medical explanation.

**misalignment** – when things go wrong. Alignment doesn't always happen, even in our everyday conversations. This can be anything from a full-scale argument to smaller moments where the talk feels a bit uncomfortable or as if you are talking at cross-purposes with the other speaker. They're not entirely desirable but, because everybody experiences these moments, they're nothing to panic about. The section on structuring and the e-learning module gives some tips on where they might happen and how to recover from them.

**quick questions** – the rapid-fire questions that you often ask in data-gathering with short, usually yes/no answers from the patient. Communication skills courses love banging on about open-ended questions, and they're great. But there's also a time and a place for rapid questions, particularly if you have a lot of clinical questions to get through and the patient gets on board and aligns with this questioning strategy.

**signposting** – is pointing ahead to things you are going to talk about, or pointing back to things you have previously said. It's a particularly clear type of metacommunication that is often talked about in communication skills. Successful candidates do it a lot – but it's important to follow through and actually talk about the things you're signposting.

**slow questions** – slowing the pace down to ask more sensitive or open-ended questions. It's not just about making them open-ended, but also the speed and manner in which you deliver them, that makes 'slow questions' an important strategy.

**stock phrases** – the phrases that we use rather repeatedly, in the CSA and in GP consultations more broadly. Computational analysis shows that some phrases crop up in the CSA all the time as everyone uses them – successful and unsuccessful candidates. But you need to be careful where you put them, so that they don't sound inappropriate or just learned by rote.

# Part I

# 1 Introduction to the CSA

*Kamila Hawthorne*

## Why does the CSA exist?

This chapter sets the scene for the Clinical Skills Assessment (CSA), explaining how it came to have its current format, how it fits with the other two main assessments in the examinations for Membership of the Royal College of General Practitioners (MRCGP), and its educational rationale.

In Chapter 2, the experience of previous candidates, suggestions for preparing and the practicalities of the exam itself are discussed. In Chapter 3, some of the unhelpful 'popular myths' about the CSA, as well as some of its 'truths' (which do help with preparation for the assessment), are examined. Taken together, this will help you develop a strategy to prepare for and pass the CSA.

### How and why was the CSA introduced, and why was it designed as a 'simulated surgery'?

The CSA is one of the three assessments introduced in October 2007 as part of the licensing examinations for MRCGP. Candidates who successfully complete all three parts can apply to the General Medical Council (GMC) (via the RCGP) for its Certificate of Completion of Training (CCT). This allows a doctor to be eligible for inclusion on the GMC's GP Register and to work independently as a general practitioner in the UK.

Prior to 2007, GP registrars applying to become GPs had to pass a different set of national assessments, known as 'Summative Assessment', in order to be able to work independently in general practice. Gaining the MRCGP was not compulsory, but was taken by many to be a mark of 'excellence' in practice.

However, both the Summative Assessment and the 'old' MRCGP (pre-2007 format) were criticised on two important issues:[1]

1   The video components of both did not test clinical examination skills – consulting skills were tested as communication skills in history taking and clinical management in the consultation, with relatively little weight given to the clinical content of the consultation. Physical examination took place off screen and out of sight of the examiners

2   The video components of both were not standardised in terms of clinical content. GP registrars spent many hours compiling their 'best' video consultations, and being

selective in this way meant that the examiners saw a highly selected set of cases that did not always reflect the range and variety of general practice.

Additionally, having two separate assessments was a significant burden to trainees. An appraisal of the methods for assessing clinical skills was undertaken by the RCGP in 2004–5, which concluded that a clinical skills assessment should follow the format of an Objective Structured Clinical Examination (OSCE), testing the integration of clinical and consulting skills, and building on the established strength of the MRCGP Simulated Surgery.[2,3]

### Recent changes to the regulation of postgraduate examinations, including the MRCGP

From 2007 as part of Modernising Medical Careers (MMC), the Postgraduate Medical Education and Training Board (PMETB) approved a single-entry scheme for UK general practice based on a 'new' compulsory MRCGP curriculum and exam, to be delivered nationally by the RCGP. (PMETB, established in 2005, was the regulator of postgraduate medical training across all specialties, and was merged into the GMC in 2010.) Before 2010 the PMETB, and since 2010 the GMC, require all royal medical colleges to include an assessment of clinical skills. The original PMETB 'Principles of Assessment', which laid out the standards and requirements of professional postgraduate examinations for all medical royal colleges, have been incorporated into the GMC's *Standards for Curricula and Assessment Systems*[4] and form the regulatory framework within which the curricula and their aligned assessments must operate.

The MRCGP now consists of three parts: the Applied Knowledge Test (AKT, currently a computer-delivered and machine-marked test of knowledge and applied knowledge), the CSA (an OSCE-style clinical examination based on the format of a 'simulated surgery' of case-based 'stations') and a Workplace-Based Assessment test (WPBA) that is formatively run by the GP registrar's educational supervisor, entered onto an ePortfolio, and summatively marked centrally by the Annual Review of Competence Progression (ARCP) panels in the Local Education and Training Boards (LETBs)/postgraduate deaneries.

*A Reference Guide for Postgraduate Specialty Training in the UK* (the 'Gold Guide 2014') sets out the agreements, as decided by all UK Departments of Health for the GP and specialty training programmes.[5] The Gold Guide provides guidance to the LETBs and deaneries on the delivery of these training programmes. The RCGP does not have responsibility for preparing or training doctors to develop the knowledge and competencies that are assessed in the MRCGP assessments, but it is responsible for devising and conducting the AKT and CSA, which are centrally administered by the Exams Department of the RCGP. It is also responsible for the framework and quality management of the WPBA, which is carried out in the LETBs and deaneries.

The three parts of the MRGCP test the ability of the trainee to work in general practice in different ways, and at different levels of application of their learning. The AKT is seen as a good test of knowledge and ability to apply knowledge, in a multi-question format that allows wide and reliable sampling across the curriculum. It tests at the lower levels of 'Miller's Triangle', a well-known framework for testing educational competency progression, in which the base of good assessments is on 'knowing' and 'knowing how'

GPs work and what they need to know.[6] The CSA, as a simulated clinical examination, tests slightly higher up the Triangle, at the level of 'showing how' to work as a GP in consultations with patients. The WPBA, as a workplace-based assessment, is at the peak of the Triangle, where candidates can demonstrate that they know what needs to be done, as well as actually doing it in an authentic, assessable setting.[7]

The AKT and CSA are developed and delivered by the RCGP Exams Department via the panel of MRCGP examiners at the RCGP headquarters in Euston, London, and the WPBA is run by the LETBs (England) and the deaneries in Scotland, Wales and Northern Ireland, with the assessments designed and outcomes quality checked by the RCGP.

### *The curriculum*

The MRCGP curriculum was developed by the RCGP Curriculum Development Group (principal author Dr Mike Deighan), and approved in 2007. It was derived from the RCGP core curriculum document *Being a General Practitioner* and set out a framework of core competency domains designed by the European Academy of Teachers in General Practice (EURACT), derived from *The European Definition of General Practice/Family Medicine* of 2005.[8] This has, over the intervening years, been simplified in its terminology, aligned with the MRCGP assessments competence framework and mapped to the GMC's *Good Medical Practice*.[9]

*Being a General Practitioner* sets out the six domains of competence that define general practice as a specialty. The MRCGP assessments competence framework is based on these six domains (Appendix I, www.rcgp.org.uk/training-exams/~/media/Files/GP-training-and-exams/Curriculum-2012/RCGP-Curriculum-blueprint-2015.ashx). This has made it possible to show clearly within the core statement which MRCGP assessment tools are used to assess the core learning outcomes.[10]

The MRCGP curriculum is divided into sections that follow on from the core curriculum statement of *Being a General Practitioner*. The full curriculum statements can be found on the RCGP website at: www.rcgp.org.uk/training-exams/gp-curriculum-overview.aspx. The core curriculum statement is followed by four 'contextual' statements that each explore particular aspects of general practice in greater depth, and 21 'clinical' statements that apply the competences in *Being a General Practitioner* to population groups or system-based conditions. Full guidance on how to use these statements in preparing for the CSA is available on the RCGP website. These are reviewed every year by the RCGP to ensure that they adapt to the ever-changing nature of general practice.

It is important that all these statements are assessed as part of the MRCGP, the blueprint of which describes when and how they are assessed to cover the curriculum. In some cases, where more than one assessment method could test a particular domain (for example 'specific problem-solving skills' can be tested in all three assessment types), this is seen as an opportunity to triangulate candidates' performance. In other cases, for example 'community orientation', only one assessment method can test the domain with validity (WPBA). WPBA tests nearly all domains of the curriculum (as it takes place in the candidates' place of work), whereas the CSA as a simulated case-based 'surgery' tests mainly those aspects of a GP's work that take place in the consulting room. On a framework of biomedical knowledge, candidates need to demonstrate problem-solving skills, a holistic patient-centred approach, showing understanding of the patient context and demonstrating professional behaviour that is in line with the GMC's *Good Medical Practice*. WPBA samples widely but at low levels of standardisation, whilst the CSA has a more focused sampling, but with high reliability. The two approaches are complementary.

The assessment blueprint (Appendix I) breaks down into the three components of the MRCGP: the Applied Knowledge Test, the Clinical Skills Assessment and the Workplace-Based Assessment. In many areas, it is possible to triangulate performance by testing knowledge, skills and attitude in more than one assessment. Between them, however, they cover the whole MRCGP curriculum map. So, for the CSA, this includes sampling from all of the 'systems-based' curriculum statements (cardiology, respiratory, gastroenterology, etc.), as well as from a full age range, aspects of patient diversity, cases that include physical examinations, and cases that have a mix of biomedical and psychosocial problems.

## How is the CSA structured?

### *Principles underpinning the CSA and its structure*

The purpose of the CSA is defined as: 'an assessment of a doctor's ability to integrate and apply appropriate clinical, professional, communication and practical skills in general practice'. It is intended to be a means of assessing a doctor's ability to synthesise and assimilate information from the patient and his or her case notes, and then to integrate and apply this with competent clinical reasoning and communication with the patient, taking into account the concerns and ideas of the patient, in a variety of clinical contexts (see Appendix I).

A GP's work centres around surgery consultations, for which fluent consulting skills are needed. Understanding the lay perspective and patients' likely expectations of health and illness, and using this understanding to negotiate behaviour change and compliance with a management plan, all add to an increased likelihood of better clinical outcomes. This communicative consulting flexibility of language and culture, with a diversity of patients, is an important skill to master in addition to biomedical knowledge and problem-solving ability. It also involves use of the knowledge of the NHS and social care systems that are an integral part of the complex consultations that take place in primary care. Many GPs see up to 40 or even more patients per day, and need to keep these skills finely tuned, as well as to be able to cope with the through-put of so many consultations and the time-limited constraints this system imposes. The GP's role as patient advocate, and initiator of the referral process, steering patients through the complexities of the NHS appointments system, is also vital to the effective management of their various presentations. As our population ages, and with the move to transfer as much patient care as possible to community settings, GPs of tomorrow need to be able to cope with the demands of efficient and skilful consulting with patients who are likely to come with complex issues, more than one problem, or with many clinical problems that interact and influence each other.

The CSA is therefore designed to replicate the activities GPs perform on a day-to-day basis in an NHS surgery, as follows:

- recognition and management of common medical conditions in primary care
- demonstrating problem-solving skills and clinical judgement in the choice of focused history taking, examination, investigations and their interpretation, and demonstration of a structured and flexible approach to decision making
- a comprehensive approach to co-morbidity and management of risk
- demonstration of person-centred care – using recognised consultation techniques to promote a shared approach with the patient
- demonstration of appropriate attitudes to the consultation, showing respect for equality and diversity, within professional codes of conduct
- demonstration of proficiency in undertaking physical examinations, using diagnostic instruments as appropriate.

The OSCE-style method of the CSA has been chosen to ensure standardisation of the clinical consultation assessment and reliability of that assessment by sufficiently wide sampling and number of independent-examiner judgements. It consists of a thirteen-station series of simulations, or 'cases', each lasting 10 minutes. The 'patient' in each case is played by a role-player, who has been trained to play the role and who understands the nature and purpose of the examination. Three circuits are run simultaneously during each day of the examination, so each role is played by three role-players at any one session, who have been calibrated together and fine-tuned at the beginning of the day to be as similar as possible in terms of the information given, response to cues and emotional affect of the role.

Candidates should bear in mind that, although the appearance is of a 'usual' surgery consultation, these cases are different because they consist of a series of 'testing competences' that have been strung together to give the appearance of a normal, authentic consultation. So, for example, the case may be written in such a way that the candidate is not encouraged to explore a particular aspect of the clinical context because it isn't part of the competencies being targeted for testing in that case. For example, a diabetic patient with depression may have excellent glycosylated haemoglobin (HbA1c) results to stop the candidate from spending time on the diabetic management, and in fact it is the management of depression that is being tested. Likewise, if a physical examination is intended to be a part of the marking for a case, the candidate is not prevented from offering and performing that examination, but if it has been decided that it is not to be tested in that case, then either the role will be written in such a way that the examination is not indicated, or the examiner will hand the candidate the clinical findings from the examination so that it does not have to be performed as part of the assessment.

The cases are written by a team of MRCGP examiners, who are all UK GPs working in the NHS (or Defence Forces as GPs) themselves. They have been trained in case writing and use a template that includes the biopsychosocial background to the case (the 'narrative'), a role-player and examiner briefing, case notes for the candidate and a case-specific marking schedule. We have emulated this style in the case notes that accompany this book. All cases in the CSA have been piloted and carefully checked to ensure they are valid and medically correct examples of UK general practice, and can be completed within the 10 minutes allocated to each 'case' in the assessment.

Each case has a specific link to learning outcomes in the MRCGP curriculum, and the case-writing team has produced cases that span the MRCGP curriculum in those domains that can be tested by the CSA methodology. A CSA testing blueprint allows selection of cases from the case bank to ensure consistent spread of cases and case difficulty from a pre-agreed range of testing areas (for example the proportion of male: female cases, number of cases that include a physical examination, number of cases that involve children or older people, diversity, or a health promotion focus). A variety of different clinical contexts are possible in the simulated setting, including telephone triage cases and home visits. It is definitely worth thinking about the possible combinations of clinical/contextual settings that might present in the CSA, bearing in mind that case writers are often writing cases from real-life situations they themselves have encountered. As UK NHS GPs, these are likely to be very similar to your own experience of patients.

### Who are the examiners and how is the CSA marked?

The examiners are all experienced practising GPs, from all areas of the UK. Most are GP principals, some are salaried GPs, some work in the Defence Forces, and some have portfolio careers. Many are also GP educational supervisors or work in senior posts in LETBs or the deaneries. They have undergone a rigorous selection process that includes taking and passing the AKT (if they originally took it more than 10 years before applying to become an examiner), and a competency-based selection process at a one-day event held at the RCGP, which measures their ability to rate clinical performance reliably, work well in teams and respond to feedback. Examiners receive ongoing training during the exam period as well as at the examiners' annual conference. This includes peer review of marking performance, reflective learning from viewing and marking video examples of cases, and annual training in equality and diversity issues.

The marking schedule is based on three marking domains that are the same for each case: Data-Gathering, Clinical Management and Interpersonal Skills. The content of each case-specific marking schedule is developed from generic statements in a generic marking schedule, based on positive and negative indicators within each domain. A generic marking scheme that is then adapted for each individual case is available on the MRCGP web page,[11] and is reproduced in Appendix II.

Examiners are trained to give grades for the three domains, with each domain grade accompanied by a description of that grade. The domain grade is an integrated global mark for performance in that domain overall, not based on a checklist of items (which tends to assess at a lower level of competence than the integrated clinical performance being sought in the CSA).[12,13]

Each domain is graded similarly, with a maximum of 3 points available for each domain (there are four grades, with 3 points for a 'clear pass', 2 points for a 'pass', 1 point for a 'fail' and 0 points for a 'clear fail'). Therefore the overall case score will be between 9 and 0 points, and the total number of marks available for the assessment overall is 117 (or 13 × 9).

Examiners also indicate at the end of their marking for a case whether they feel the candidate's performance has been passing, borderline or failing, and this indication is fed into the standard-setting process to set the pass mark for the day, which uses a 'borderline standard setting' method that is well accepted for OSCE-style assessments.[14] The purpose of standard setting is to provide equivalence between one assessment and another. For example, factors such as the rarity of a condition, the emotional affect of a case, or merely adding in a requirement for a physical examination can all add 'difficulty' to the cases, and these will vary according to the selection of cases for each day. Using a standard-setting method in addition to selecting cases according to an assessment blueprint help each day's exam to be of reasonable equivalence in terms of difficulty from day to day. This is why the pass mark can vary slightly from one day to the next.

Finally, examiners indicate which, if any, of the 16 generic Feedback Statements apply to the performance of the case they have just marked. See Chapter 3 to learn more about how to use the Feedback Statements constructively and proactively. Feedback Statements are revised periodically, and so candidates are advised to look them up on the CSA web pages, where there is information on how to use them.

### References

1. Munro N, Hawthorne K, Denney ML, *et al*. Developing a new clinical skills assessment (CSA) for licensing general practitioners; the why, the how and the when. *Education for Primary Care* 2006; **17(4)**: 354–61.
2. Burrows PJ, Bingham L. The simulated surgery – an alternative to videotape submission for the consulting skills component of the MRCGP examination: the first year's experience. *British Journal of General Practice* 1999; **49(44)**: 269–72.
3. Thomas H, Field S, Hibble A, *et al*. *Training Curriculum. Submission to: Postgraduate Medical Education and Training Board*. London: RCGP, 2005. www.rcgp.org.uk/training-exams/~/media/Files/GP-training-and-exams/Curriculum%20other%20docs/curr_PMETB_06_The_Training_Curriculum.ashx [accessed 22 January 2015].
4. General Medical Council *Standards for Curricula and Assessment Systems*. Manchester: GMC, 2010. www.gmc-uk.org/Standards_for_curricula_and_assessment_systems_1114.pdf_48904896.pdf [accessed 22 January 2015].
5. *A Reference Guide for Postgraduate Specialty Training in the UK* ('The Gold Guide'). 5th edn. 2014. http://specialtytraining.hee.nhs.uk/files/2013/10/A-Reference-Guide-for-Postgraduate-Specialty-Training-in-the-UK.pdf [accessed 22 January 2015].
6. Miller GE. The assessment of clinical skills/competence/performance. *Academic Medicine* 1990; **65(9)**: S63–7.
7. Schuwirth LW, van der Vleuten CP. The use of clinical simulations in assessment. *Medical Education* 2003; **37(Suppl 1)**: 65–71.
8. European Academy of Teachers in General Practice. *The European Definition of General Practice/Family Medicine*. Euract, 2005. www.woncaeurope.org/sites/default/files/documents/Definition%20EURACTshort%20version.pdf [accessed 25 March 2015].
9. General Medical Council. *Good Medical Practice*. Manchester: GMC, 2013. www.gmc-uk.org/static/documents/content/Good_medical_practice_-_English_0914.pdf [accessed 22 January 2015].
10. Dr Ben Riley, Director of MRCGP Curriculum Development Group, personal communication, January 2015.
11. RCGP generic marking schedule. www.rcgp.org.uk/gp-training-and-exams/mrcgp-exams-overview/~/media/BD43B1D830F14793A92C505360F50D08.ashx [accessed 22 January 2015].
12. Regehr G, MacRae H, Reznick RK, Szalay D. Comparing the psychometric properties of checklists and global rating scales for assessing performance on an OSCE format examination. *Academic Medicine* 1998; **73(9)**: 993–7.
13. Hodges B, Regehr G, McNaughton N, *et al*. OSCE checklists do not capture increasing levels of expertise. *Academic Medicine* 1999; **74(10)**: 1129–34.
14. Cizek GJ, Bunch MB. The contrasting groups and borderline group methods. In: *Standard Setting*. Thousand Oaks, CA: Sage, 2007, pp. 105–13.

# 2 Preparing for the CSA

*Alexandra Rolfe and Kamila Hawthorne*

## Information and tips on preparation

The Clinical Skills Assessment (CSA) is an important element of GP training so it is worth investing time in preparing well. The CSA can only be taken during the ST3 stage of training and advisedly after spending at least six months in general practice. Clinical experience, and reflecting on your consultation skills, are the main forms of preparation so make sure you see plenty of patients with a wide variety of presentations, both acute and chronic. As the CSA allows 10 minutes per case you should ideally be competent in 10-minute consultations before the exam.

However, although similar, the CSA is not the same as your day job. You will be observed and marked so you need to ensure that the examiner knows what you are thinking and doing, and you need to get used to the idea of being watched. This may mean that you need to use additional communication measures above and beyond those used in day-to-day consulting. For example, a role-player may ask for details about what you are doing and why. Most patients don't ask questions like: 'Why do you want to examine my chest?' By using these slightly unusual questions for a patient, the role-player is helping you ensure that you have both a sensible plan of action, and have verbalised it, before the examiner lets you carry on with the physical examination or offers you a card with examination findings on it (this is done to save time in a 10-minute station so that other areas of the consultation can be focused on). Role-players ask these questions to help you indicate your thought processes, so don't feel put off by them. Communication methods and skills will be discussed in much greater depth in Chapters 4 and 5.

As most trainees do substantial further preparation this chapter will suggest ideas on how to prepare and give tips on the exam itself.

### Preparing for the exam

Ideally, sit the Applied Knowledge Test (AKT) first. The most common causes of failure in the CSA are in the Clinical Management domain and the Interpersonal Skills domain. If you pass the AKT well your knowledge is at the level required for the CSA. If you have sat the AKT recently and done well, don't spend too much time on specifics and guidelines – focus more on the consultation itself. You do not have to be an expert in everything, but you must know what to do when you don't know what to do! A good learning resource for the exam is the *Oxford Handbook of General Practice* as this gives an outline of many of the problems a GP will face.

Consider starting to prepare for the CSA at least three months before the exam, especially if you have substantial commitments outside work such as childcare. Many of the consulting habits you learn now will stand you in good stead for the rest of your clinical career.

Although clinical experience is essential, it is impossible to cover all possible presentations so further practice in small groups is highly recommended. You may practise in small groups as part of a vocational training programme, but if possible arrange to meet up in-between. If you are struggling to find a group – perhaps you are new to the area, live quite far from where you work or are sitting the exam at a less popular time – ask around or ask your local deanery/Local Education and Training Board (LETB) for advice. Sometimes it is better to study with people who you are not as familiar with as you will most likely be more focused on the topic and receive more objective feedback. Consider having more than one study group so that you can practise with different people and aim to meet with your group(s) one or two times per week.

If possible, you should have at least three members in your group – this will allow for a doctor, a role-player and an observer. Practise a wide variety of consultations from varied sources, such as patients you see in practice, cases from study books or trainee websites. However, none of these is a substitute for making up your own cases as you will gain an insight into the structure of cases, what is feasible in 10 minutes and, importantly, how the cases are marked. Some deaneries/LETBs employ actors for CSA practice; this is very useful as it will help you understand what a CSA patient may be like. It is a very good idea to video a number of consultations to see how you come across to others and observe your behaviours more closely – many candidates have told us that this was very helpful in realising what they did well, and what they did badly, especially if they watched themselves with a 'critical friend' such as another GP registrar or their educational supervisor. There may be a number of things that you don't realise you are doing. Further guidance on designing and assessing consultations can be found in Chapters 4 and 5.

### Practising the consultation

The CSA is all about the consultation so initially it is worth thinking about how you structure your consultation to include all the components required – Data-Gathering, Clinical Management and Interpersonal Skills. This chapter gives an overview of the consultation and Chapters 4 and 5 focus on various components of the consultation and communication techniques that are employed by stronger candidates.

It may be useful to have a working knowledge of a consultation model to help you structure your consultation and be a guide if things start to go wrong. However, it is very important that you are able to adapt your consultation to suit the needs of the role-player and do not stick rigidly to one model – as you know, not all types of consultation are the same and one consultation model won't apply to every situation. For example, there are times when you need to be doctor-centred and times when you should be patient-centred. So be prepared to vary your consultation structure, otherwise you could end up looking very stylised or formulaic. Some of the concepts developed in Chapters 4 and 5 do not belong to a recognised model, but come from recent sociolinguistic analysis of real CSA cases, and you may find it useful to incorporate them into your personal consulting style.

> **TIP** – There is nothing to stop you from briefly writing down a consultation structure from memory on the whiteboard in the CSA room as soon as you get in there and checking it if you get stuck.

Practise your flexible consultation style with patients in practice and in your study group so that you are very comfortable with it. This will help prevent you sounding scripted and hopefully allow you to get back on track if it feels as if things are going wrong. Start with open questions and allow the patient time to speak. Make sure you listen to the patient and respond actively to what he or she says, and try not to ask the same question repeatedly. Have a sensible way of asking about ideas, concerns and expectations, and do not close your questions too quickly. If you are addressing sensitive areas let the patient know this is happening. Use your own words to ask questions, not the suggested phrases in the textbooks. This will make you sound more natural. Make sure that you are responding sensibly and logically to the patient and signpost changes of subject so that the patient (and examiner in the CSA exam) can follow your train of thought.

Once you have the finished the data-gathering, if appropriate, make a sensible diagnosis and explain it to the patient in a way he or she can understand. Consider how this diagnosis will affect the patient's life.

> **TIP** – Make a diagnosis if there is one – you may lose marks for not committing to a possible diagnosis when it is straightforward.

To help, consider practising the explanation of specific topics/diagnoses in lay terms. Perhaps try to keep a list of the patients you see on a day-to-day basis, and their diagnoses, and practise explaining those diagnoses. For example, how would you describe hypothyroidism or coronary artery disease in an understandable way? You don't want to be doing this for the first time in the CSA! Perhaps use non-medical family and friends to practise on and case-cards can be very useful. Additionally, work out a strategy for what to do when you do not know the answer/diagnosis – what would you do and what would you tell the patient? Remember that GPs as generalists are not expected to know everything.

If appropriate, examine the patient. Good, focused clinical examinations are an important part of general practice and therefore also the CSA, and they are becoming more common. Make sure you practise them and have a familiarity with the equipment required. There is also the possibility that models could be used for more intimate examinations. Don't forget about the less common examinations such as visual acuity and visual fields – it is not good enough just to suggest a visit to the optician. Be able to use a Snellen chart and tuning forks for limb sensation and Weber's and Rinne's tests. The RCGP website contains a list of equipment to bring, but remember other equipment may appear on the desk for you to use.

Then, as appropriate, discuss management options with the patient/carer. There are a number of ways to conduct this part of the consultation and don't be afraid to 'guide' the patient. You could be directive and tell the patient what the best option is; you could allow the patient control and let the patient choose the management he or she wants; or you could offer the options and then guide the patient. The last approach is often the most effective, but does depend on the nature of the consultation. For example – 'I think that it is this … so we could do this investigation or treat it like this.' Remember, there is nothing stopping the patient from going away and thinking about it and then coming back. In the exam itself, use your BNF as appropriate and be aware that, if you give the role-player a prescription, he or she will take it out of the room and the examiner will be given it and will mark it, so make sure it is correct! But don't spend too long reading the BNF! It is acceptable to put in chapter markers in the BNF, although you can't of course write anything in it. Taking a children's BNF is also a requirement.

> **TIP** – If you write a prescription, read it out to the patient while showing it to him or her. This is a good part of everyday practice and it also makes it less likely that you will make a mistake. It is possible that you might have to write a controlled drug prescription, so make sure you know how to do it accurately. In the CSA itself, if you give a prescription to the patient (and some cases do require this), it will be seen by the examiner and marked for clinical accuracy and appropriateness.

If you do not know the diagnosis or the patient asks a question that you do not know the answer to, be honest rather than make something up. You can tell the patient that you will look it up and then get back to him or her later.

Throughout the consultation, check understanding by using your own words in a sensitive way, not by asking 'How will you explain this to your wife/husband etc.?' or other phrases suggested by the books. Use your own – it will sound so much more natural! If you wish to suggest an information sheet this is OK, but you must explain what it will say. Otherwise, the examiner can't mark your knowledge. Signposting patients to websites can also be useful, such as to the British Heart Foundation, www.patient.co.uk, etc., but be familiar with them. You could write down a website and name of a condition for the patient to refer to later.

There are a number of scenarios that you need to consider. You should be prepared for a number of ethical dilemmas in the case mix. These are often the hardest cases for you to deal with as there may not be a correct answer. The important thing is to take a good history, address any major concerns – e.g. a child protection issue – and find out what the role-player thinks and wants to know or do. You may disagree with the role-player, but you must explain why. Don't try to second-guess what you think the examiner will want you to say because you can tie yourself up in knots doing this – it's much better to be yourself and say what you think is right. Second, on occasions there may be a home visit or telephone consultation. Make sure you practise these and are not thrown by them during the exam. The floor marshals will take you to and from home visits, and tell you what you need to take into the room, so you don't need to worry about anything except what happens during the case itself.

In your study group practise, time your consultations, and stop at 10 minutes. Then, using the CSA guide, mark the consultation. Mark the doctor quite critically – be fair, but not necessarily too nice just because you like the person. Now is the time to improve, not after the exam. When giving feedback to the doctor start with a positive, then discuss any improvements that could be made. If possible, try to do this in a constructive way, such as, 'You did this … but you could do this.'

Initially just practise a couple of consultations each; as you progress you will find that you can get through more, but the quality is much more important than the quantity. Remember to include a good variety of backgrounds, cultures, etc. in your cases.

Further information about aspects of the consultation that are demonstrated by strong candidates can be found in Chapters 4 and 5. A number of practice cases and guidance on how to make up your own cases are found in Part II.

Many candidates worry excessively about taking the CSA component of the MRCGP. Build up your self-esteem and confidence in your abilities as a good consulter. One of the best ways to do this is by getting a lot of practice seeing as many patients as you can in a similar consulting environment (you can see this from the video introduction to the assessment centre on the MRCGP web page). Ask your study colleagues and your trainer to watch video consultations and critique them, and watch them and mark them yourself using adaptations of the marking schedule examples in this book. Also prepare by thinking of the assessment as 'just another surgery' – you will find that the role-player patients are so well trained that you can quickly imagine they are real.

If you work in an area where most of your patients consult with you in a language that is not English, or need an interpreter, then ask your educational supervisor/trainer and programme director to find you a practice where you can see patients who consult in English as part of your preparation for the CSA. Doing some surgeries there will be invaluable for 'getting you into the mindset' of the CSA.

Finally, many trainees ask if they should go on a course. This is an individual decision and will depend on how you like to learn and prepare for examinations. Hopefully, your training scheme will have put on a formative CSA – even running through a few cases is helpful and getting feedback on your performance from your peers or educational supervisors can help you work out your strengths and weaknesses. Many candidates, however, say that going on courses has not really helped them, so you should not feel that this is mandatory.

## The exam itself

### Getting to the exam

As soon as you book your exam via the RCGP website, which details the dates of the exam and the booking procedure, arrange your accommodation and travel. The RCGP website lists suitable local accommodation. You will not be able to stay at the RCGP headquarters, as the examiners will be there. Stay close by and, if you have a morning exam or are coming from far away, arrive the night before. Sometimes weather conditions can cause delays, so factor this possibility into your timings, especially if you are coming during the winter. The exam centre is very close to both Euston and King's Cross stations so is easy to get to. It can be nice to take someone with you for moral support such as your partner, and this is especially helpful if they are non-medical. If you are thinking about travelling with your peers who are also sitting the exam, be careful, as this could put more pressure on you as they may make you feel underprepared. After the exam they could increase your anxiety about the exam because of differing answers that you might have given.

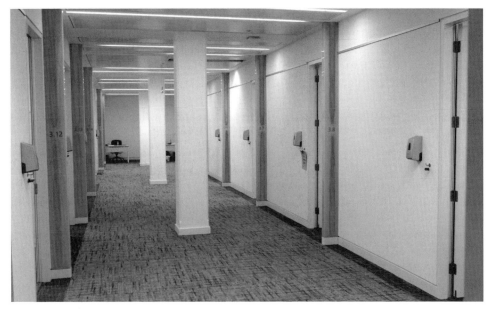

*Figure 2.1* The exam centre

### On the day

A good breakfast is most important, and don't overdo the coffee! Make sure you have all the required equipment and suitable clothes – the majority of trainees wear suits, both male and female, but make sure that you are comfortable. It is important to look smart to show that you are taking the exam seriously. There is a dress code on the RCGP website.

Familiarise yourself with the location of the RCGP. The exam entrance is around the corner from the main entrance and the exam circuit itself. A very good video walkthrough of the exam, made by *GP* magazine, can be found on the RCGP website. There are three circuits that can run concurrently.

You will arrive quite a while before the exam, especially if you are in the afternoon. You are then ushered into a room where you all wait until you are ready for the exam briefing – this could be up to one hour, but tea and coffee and biscuits are laid on. The exam briefing is led by the senior marshal for the day, an experienced examiner, and you are free to ask any last-minute questions. It is short, about 15–20 minutes, and is aimed to keep you calm and informed about what is going to happen when you get to the circuits.

Use this time carefully – if you like last-minute revising you can read, or you can sit and stare into space, or chat to other candidates but be careful not to let them make you more anxious. You will then be taken to your room and given 10–15 minutes in which to unpack your bags, lock away anything you don't need for the exam and get settled in. The rooms vary: some have no windows; some are next to a main road. Although there is noise reduction it is not completely silent – but neither is a normal consulting room! Be aware of this and do not let it distract you. Have a look at what is on the desk and think about how you might use it, e.g. tuning forks, peak flow, etc., and lay your equipment on the desk. There will also be an iPad on the desk with an RCGP app. There is, of course, no access to other programmes, or to the internet. The iPad will contain information about the cases. Although you are able to read all the cases, make sure that you are on the correct case. The RCGP website has a guide to the use of iPads in the CSA for candidates, and it is very easy to use.

### The exam

Take a deep breath, relax and think of it as a normal surgery, but without the admin, phone interruptions and IT. Read the notes on the first role-player; the buzzer will sound and someone will knock on the door. Call them in and go to the door if they do not enter – this may be a subtle sign. There will be at least two people at the door: the role-player and the examiner. Do not be surprised if there are more. There may be another examiner (who is there to quality-assure the process) or carer for the role-player. There may be a child role-player with their parent/carer. The examiner will usually sit away from your line of sight – ignore him or her.

Shake the role-player patient by the hand (if this is what you are comfortable doing), introduce yourself, welcome him or her in – clues may come from this – and start your consultation. Follow your routine and try hard to cover the three domains of the CSA. There is a digital clock on the wall that counts up the 10 minutes which you have for the case. At the end of 10 minutes the buzzer will go and the role-player and examiner will leave. This could be in the middle of a sentence. Don't worry about this – they are only doing what they have been told to do, and it's necessary for the circuits to keep to time. They will not usually give much away so a stony-faced role-player does not mean you have failed. After each case remember Roger Neighbour's 'housekeeping' concept: it is very important to forget about the last case and move on to the next one.[1] You can easily do badly on one case and still pass the exam well, but this is less likely if you dwell on what might have gone wrong.

> **TIP** – The role-player does not have to have left the room by the end of the consultation. As long as you have covered the three domains well, you will still get your marks.

Don't forget home visits and telephone consultations, and do not be put off by them. Follow the instructions that you are given. For a telephone encounter there will be a role-player on the other end of the phone in your room and an examiner listening in. For a home visit someone will come to get you and then escort you back to your room afterwards.

Some cases require a physical examination. Proceed as you would for a patient you were seeing in your own surgery. Offer the examination, offer a chaperone if needed, and explain what you want to do and why. Sometimes, at this point, the examiner will offer you a card with the examination findings on it or give verbal findings. Accept the findings and move on with the consultation. If you are not offered a card with findings on it, this means that you are expected to carry out the examination you have proposed. All consulting rooms in the CSA circuits have examination couches, and any additional clinical equipment over and above that you have been requested to bring with you will be provided.

There will be 13 cases with a two-minute break between them and then a longer break in the middle (after seven cases), when you are allowed to stretch your legs, visit the bathroom, and have a drink and a biscuit.

After the last case, once all materials and papers have been gathered in and your belongings returned to you, you are allowed to leave. This is when you need your non-GP friends; try not to discuss the exam, because this will inevitably make you feel bad and that you have messed things up. You are bound to want to discuss the exam at length with your trainer. But remember, you cannot turn back the clock, and you have given your written promise not to discuss CSA cases with others. You may feel that you missed the point of a case, but if you looked for a hidden agenda and were not given anything, there probably wasn't one. Try to do something completely different and wait for the results.

The results will be put straight into your ePortfolio on a predetermined date and will contain feedback if the same Feedback Statement has been ticked at least twice.

Hopefully, you will find that the preparation for taking the CSA makes a big difference to your everyday consultations and makes you a better doctor.

### Key points

- Start preparing for the exam well in advance.
- Be on 10-minute appointments before the exam.
- Practise in groups – more than one is ideal.
- Use non-medical people to practise on.
- Use a combination of prepared and self-made practice cases.
- Think about how to manipulate the consultation to ensure the examiner knows what you are doing and why.

### Reference

1. Neighbour R. *The Inner Consultation: How to Develop an Effective and Intuitive Consulting Style.* 2nd edn. Abingdon: Radcliffe Publishing, 2005.

# 3  Myths and truths about the CSA

*Kamila Hawthorne*

## Myths

There are a number of popular myths about the Clinical Skills Assessment (CSA) that need to be dispelled before you can start really preparing. These include the following.

1  'It is a test of your ability to act, rather than a test of knowledge, clinical skills or consulting acumen.' As many doctors will agree, a lot of consulting is about putting on an 'act' – to give confidence to the patient as well as to set the basis for that doctor/patient relationship that is so important to good outcomes. But the CSA is NOT a test of acting ability in addition to what you would normally do in a consultation. It DOES require you to put aside your anxiety about the exam, to forget where you are, and concentrate on the person in front of you. We know from candidate exit surveys that nearly all candidates find the role-players so convincing that they can't believe

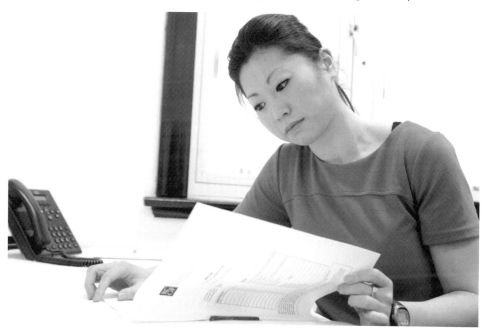

*Figure 3.1* A candidate prepares for the CSA

they are not being faced with a real patient. This is a necessary requirement of any simulated clinical examination in any medical specialty.

2  'The role-players will decide whether you pass or fail, and can be biased in their judgements.' There have been a number of studies of role-player behaviour in the CSA, which have not found any evidence of bias in role-player behaviour.[1,2] The Knowledge Transfer Partnership is a sociolinguistic research project funded by the Technology Strategy Board and the Academy of Medical Royal Colleges, and in partnership with the RCGP, King's College London and Cardiff University. It looked at a small number of cases in great detail, analysing the nature of the talking between the role-player patients and the candidates. It found no evidence of role-player patient bias in any of the cases researched. Its findings are discussed in detail in Chapter 4. As described earlier, the role-players play no part in marking decisions in the CSA.

3  'The examiners can be biased in their judgements.' There have been a number of studies (both quantitative and qualitative) made on examiner behaviour in marking, and no evidence has been found for this statement.[3] A Judicial Review brought by the British Association of Physicians of Indian Origin (BAPIO) in April 2014 decided that there was no evidence of either direct or indirect discrimination in the CSA, or that the RCGP had not fulfilled its Public Sector Equality Duty (PSED) in relation to the differential pass rates noted for International Medical Graduates, compared with UK graduates.

4  'The cases don't reflect "real-life" general practice.' Some of the aspects of the simulation have been described in previous chapters but within the limitations of the assessment method many candidates tell us that they find the cases to be very realistic and that the role-players playing these roles seem just like real patients. There are difficulties in portraying every type of case you might find in general practice, as well as simulating the regional differences between patients. Some types of patient cannot be simulated in the CSA – for example patients who don't speak English (it would take too long if an interpreter was also incorporated into the consultation), babies and roles that required an intimate examination. However, the cases are written by practising GPs, are quality assured by other GPs and are piloted carefully, with amendments and changes made to ensure the case is as real as possible before it is used in an examination circuit. Cases are also updated regularly, to keep in line with current medical practice.

## Truths

There are also some truths about the CSA that need to be taken into account when preparing for this examination. These include the following.

1  There are some aspects of the MRCGP curriculum that are very difficult or impossible to simulate in a CSA setting (see above). This means that, if you are preparing for the CSA, you can work out some types of case that are very unlikely to appear and concentrate on those you think are likely to appear. This includes areas where there are significant regional differences, such as those relating to the Mental Health Act. Bear in mind, though, that the examiner case writers are very resourceful and may think up a way to include them after all. ...

2   As all the role-players are 'well' there won't be any 'real' clinical signs to pick up in an examination. The converse is that, if you do pick up a clinical sign, you may have to work out if it is relevant to the case or not. Role-players requiring a physical examination have already been checked by the examiner working with them for that day, and so all such 'red herrings' should have been found and excluded.

3   You will have to perform clinical examinations, despite knowing that it is very unlikely you will pick up abnormal clinical signs. Therefore you must practise doing these clinical examinations. It is important that those physical examinations you do are done confidently and in line with expected practice, such that the examiner can feel that you would have picked up abnormal signs if there were any there to find.

4   You will need to make sure the examiner knows how you are thinking and developing your diagnosis and clinical management for the case, which means that you will need to go a step further than you may normally do in real life, in ensuring he or she knows what you are doing:

   a   Make sure you explain what you are doing to the patient, and what you find if you are examining the patient – this is good practice anyway, but you may need to take more trouble doing this so that the examiner knows what you are thinking

   b   Make sure you explain your management to the patient – even more than you would normally do. Role-players help candidates by asking what suggested examinations and tests are for, which real patients tend not to do!

5   You need to be very aware of the role-player, and listen actively to what he or she says. The role-player may give you cues that bring you back on track if you are digressing into an area that is not being marked by the case. If the role-player appears to shut you down, be aware that he or she may be helping you by indicating you need to explore a different course of questions or enquiry. He or she may also drop cues or hints, or ask questions that help you find the right track more easily, if you are listening and pick them up.

6   Use the guidance and tips that are on the MRCGP CSA web pages. Many candidates don't seem to know these are there and that there is a lot of information freely available. This includes:

   a   A video 'walkthrough' of the CSA Assessment Centre

   b   The MRCGP curriculum

   c   Guidance on the CSA and how to prepare

   d   How cases are constructed

   e   The Generic Marking Schedule

   f   How to use the Feedback Statements. It may seem counter-intuitive, but they do say that 'wise men learn from other people's mistakes'! So please do look at the explanation for each Feedback Statement and the tips to improve that accompany each Feedback Statement. There are currently 16 Feedback Statements, in four categories: general comments about overall consulting style, as well as more specific comments in each of the three marking domains of Data-Gathering, Clinical Management and Interpersonal Skills. Candidates currently receive Feedback Statements that have been ticked by examiners two or more times during their CSA. But you can learn a lot from the detailed explanations for each statement, even if you have not yet taken the examination, and use the tips to improve in your preparation.

### References

1. Russell D, Etherington C, Hawthorne K. How can simulated patients' experiences suggest ways to improve candidate performance in the MRCGP clinical assessments? *Education for Primary Care* 2012; **23(6)**: 391–8.
2. Foreman P, Hawthorne K. The effects of role player-candidate interactions on fairness in the CSA. AMEE Conference 2013. http://ieposter.com/eposter_manager/modules/eposter/templates/preview_eposter.php?key=TVRFNVhsNWVNamd6WGw1ZU1qZ3o= [accessed 22 January 2015].
3. Denney ML, Freeman A, Wakeford R. MRCGP CSA: are the examiners biased, favouring their own by sex, ethnicity and degree source? *British Journal of General Practice* 2013; DOI: 10.3399/bjgp13X674396.

# 4 Structure and alignment in the CSA consultation

*Sarah Atkins and Celia Roberts*

## Thinking about what makes good 'talk'

The Clinical Skills Assessment (CSA) is all about putting your clinical knowledge into action. You'll already know, from working as a GP, that being able to discover the right information about the patient and communicate information effectively is a vitally important skill. In fact it's probably the main work you do day in, day out. Much of this important work in the consultation is done through *talk*.

The CSA tests some of these skills, although of course it can't test every aspect of day-to-day GP life. The CSA can examine particular competences that are very important to general practice, particularly in relation to your consultation skills. These are features such as being able to structure your data-gathering and clinical management in a logical order, give good explanations of diagnostic decisions or treatment plans and being able to talk in partnership with a role-played patient. These are the kind of features that we'll give tips on in this chapter. However, these tips do not form a recipe-like list of instructions for how to carry out your CSA consultations. We give some hints and ideas for things you can try out, but it's also important to find your own style of consulting that you feel comfortable with. We know there is no 'one size fits all' consultation style, and that's as true for GPs themselves as it is for patients.

Some of these ideas might also seem familiar – after all, you have been carrying out real consultations with patients for years and you already know many useful strategies. Sometimes, though, it can be helpful to tease out and highlight what those communication skills are, so that you can think about them in preparation for an exam. Because it can take some time to try out strategies and find a consultation style you are comfortable with, we'd suggest looking at the ideas in this chapter and discussing them with your GP trainer and colleagues throughout your training. Nevertheless, even if you're reading this a few weeks from your CSA there are still lots of ideas you can take on board, which build on all the things you will have already learned about conducting consultations. While the chapter gives tips designed for trainees preparing for the CSA, we hope it also gives some ideas for thinking about 'talk' in general practice that are useful beyond the assessment.

### Where do these ideas come from?

The ideas outlined in this chapter come directly from the findings of a research project (Roberts, Atkins and Hawthorne, 2014) that carefully analysed videos of candidates sitting the CSA.[1] This research looked at equal numbers of passing and failing candidates, of all different backgrounds, to establish if there are any communicative features that contribute to success or failure. This chapter presents those findings in terms of practical tips for how 'talk' works in the exam, particularly areas where candidates did well or badly when interacting with role-played patients.

In order to be specific about the findings of the research, as well as give a fresh look at the consultation, we have borrowed a few words from the field of linguistics. You might therefore encounter some terminology that is new to you, but we hope this makes the chapter more interesting and insightful. These new terms can be referred to in the glossary (see pp. xv–xvi).

In presenting these findings in a practical guide, we've also kept in mind some of the previous literature on healthcare communication. There is a whole host of communication skills literature in medicine that you might have encountered during your undergraduate and postgraduate training. We'll pick up on some ideas from classic guides like the Calgary–Cambridge model[2] and Roger Neighbour's *The Inner Consultation*,[3] which you might well have encountered during your medical training. However, much more importantly we also look at where models can go wrong and ideas for managing some of the messier realities of real-time talk. It's important to think about how you employ models and the occasions that need a bit of flexibility. Real talk is naturally 'messier' than it looks in communication models. But if you look at evidence of the actual talk, as we'll do in this chapter, it's possible to see that there's still a systematic organisation to all this apparently 'messy' talk. Understanding how messy real talk works can often be much more helpful than a scripted communication skills model. We can only really understand the complexities of this 'real talk' by looking at real language data.

### 'Real' data from simulated cases

The research was all about looking at real CSA talk – not what we think might happen, but what actually happens in the exam. So that you can see what happens 'inside the CSA', this chapter presents some transcripts of talk taken directly from the exam. This means you can see, for real, how candidates handle the various role-plays. Of course, it's not 'real-life' talk in the sense that it comes from real GP surgeries – this is still a simulated, Objective Structured Clinical Examination (OSCE)-style exam after all. However, these transcripts are authentic in that they show genuine GP candidates who are taking the exam, all for the first time, who clearly have a very real stake in doing well. Seeing what they do can give you some ideas of what the exam is like. It also demonstrates that you don't have to sound like a 'perfect' communication skills robot to manage the CSA consultations well.

Try to keep in mind what we've said about the messiness of 'real talk' – false starts and hesitations are all part of how real-time talk works, even outside stressful exam settings. These candidates would be the first to point out that they don't do everything perfectly. So be kind to the candidates you're about to look at – they've been nice enough to let you read extracts of their talk and see footage from their exam in the online materials. When you look closely, it's possible to see the strategies the successful candidates use to do the talking work of the consultation well. You don't have to copy these ways of talking – this chapter is not designed to be a list of recipe-like instructions but rather to help you develop and build on strategies you have already learned during your training.

Because we're using transcribed excerpts from real candidates, you're going to see actual exam cases. You won't get the same cases in your own CSA – all the cases that appear here have been suspended. They're representative of the types of cases that appear, but your exam will not be exactly the same. We've also tried to show a good range of case types, from the very routine to the quite complex. In doing so, we've shown a few of the harder cases that can come up in the CSA, in terms of the communication skills they require, but you should remember that these will not make up the majority of the cases you'll see. More importantly though, the skills we are presenting are generalisable across most case types. These are skills that were shown to be indicative of high performance or identified as an area of difficulty for many of the failing candidates. Complex cases can be pretty useful to try out for developing your communication style, but remember to practise on the more routine case types too.

### Transcripts

Looking closely at talk is what this chapter is all about. The linguists who did the research made transcripts of consented CSA candidates, so that they could examine the talk carefully. Transcripts in linguistics don't use capitals and standard punctuation marks because that isn't how we talk. So you'll see transcripts that look like this:

```
CAN:    um (.) which I understand is what your father suffered from
```

The transcripts have been simplified a little from the originals, but some notation is still helpful (see Table 4.1).

Transcripts in linguistics also mark every false start and every repeated word, and all the 'ums' and 'ahs' we produce when talking. It's useful to see this, not only from the point of view of applied linguistics, where we want to evidence claims with real data, but also from a communication skills perspective, so that we can see it's not necessary to sound completely perfect.

Transcripts mean that you can look at videos of talk in 'slow motion' and see more precisely how the talk works. We hope the tools from this course will be especially useful if you are looking at videos of your own consultations. As observing your consultations is already part of the Workplace-Based Assessment component of the MRCGP you may want to use the ideas from this book in conjunction with the RCGP's consultation observation

*Table 4.1*  Transcripts key

| | |
|---|---|
| CAN | Candidate's talk |
| RPL | Role-player's talk |
| EXM | Examiner's talk |
| (.) | Very short pauses, less than 0.5 of a second |
| (pause) | Longer pauses |
| PPP | Pausing |
| t- | Syllable cut off due to false start |
| e::: | Extended word or syllable |
| \ | Downward intonation |
| [ ] | Overlapping speech: |
| [ ] | CAN:    and then [event]ually |
| | RPL:            [yeah] |
| **** | Word blanked out – either inaudible or anonymised |

tool,[4] when discussing your consultations with your trainer. You probably don't have time to transcribe your own consultations, although it can be a useful thing to do.

Of course, while the transcripts are from real life, reading them can sometimes feel very removed from the contexts in which they were originally recorded. We'd suggest, therefore, that you use this book in conjunction with the online module available to all on the RCGP website. The module has **videos of successful candidates** – some of whom you will see the transcripts for here. Using the book in conjunction with the videos can therefore help bring some of these transcripts to life.[5]

## Key concept: 'Alignment'

Whenever we talk, be it casual conversation between our friends or more professional interactions with colleagues, we're generally trying to establish a shared understanding of what we're doing and what's being said. Linguists and philosophers have argued for centuries about how achievable this is. Nevertheless we can evidence, by looking at lots of real talk, the practical strategies people use to try to create a shared, common understanding of topics and tasks, even if it's not quite perfect.

Creating shared understanding is particularly important in professional interactions with patients. The GP and patient have a task to perform – a consultation – and must talk together to achieve it. We're going to call this process of working towards a mutual purpose through talk 'alignment'. We've chosen this word for a reason. 'Alignment' in linguistics means a level of cooperation and understanding between speakers that allows the talk to work. But it doesn't mean that you always have to like each other or agree on everything. Sometimes you might, but in most professional contexts there are usually some constraints that make this difficult. What makes 'alignment' a useful idea, then, is that it doesn't have to mean you approve wholeheartedly of someone else's world view. However, you can still both conduct the talk professionally, giving one another turns at talk and having a tacit level of agreement about the tasks being performed – data-gathering, physical examination, explanations, discussion of action plan, etc. Even in cases where the patient is angry or sticks to a very difficult moral position ('Complex cases'), you can still conduct the consultation in a way that everyone has space to talk, feels understood and can understand what is being discussed.

If this seems like a difficult idea to pin down, think about those awkward moments that we've all experienced where things go wrong and we seem to be talking at cross-purposes. This happens in our everyday conversations just as it does in GP surgeries. At these moments, 'alignment' seems to have disappeared. Now think about all the strategies you used to get things back on track. Getting things back on track and talking toward a joint purpose is 'alignment'. Keep these alignment ideas in mind as we move through the chapter.

---

### Exercise – Alignment

Write down the most recent misunderstanding you had with a patient. How did you repair this and get things back on track so that the talk was 'aligned' again? What kind of problem was the patient presenting? Can you think of a consultation where you managed to avoid difficult moments altogether?

*Table 4.2* Phases of the GP consultation

| I | **Opening** | |
|---|---|---|
| II | **Data-gathering** | |
| III | **Physical examination** | |
| IV | **Explanation** | The doctor and/or patient consider the condition (we will label this the 'Explanation' phase). |
| V | **Treatment** | The doctor and patient agree and detail further treatment or investigation if necessary |
| VI | **Closing** | |

*Source:* adapted from Byrne and Long's (1976) six phases of the consultation[6] and Heritage and Maynard (2006).[7]

## Structuring the consultation

### *Routine case structures*

In Chapter 2, we introduced a few ideas on structuring consultations. The 'structure' of a consultation here refers to the broad sequence of different tasks that comprise the whole. In Chapter 1, a rough structure was discussed. This task-based model is often seen as a doctor-centred perspective on the consultation. However, evidence seems to show that patients come to the consultation with a very similar set of tasks in mind. Achieving them actually requires a level of tacit agreement between doctor and patient about the work to be done – the kind of 'aligned' talk described above. Nevertheless, it's important to employ these task-based models with some care. Let's explore this structuring idea a little further and think about employing it strategically, rather than a rigid 'one size fits all' model. Keeping an idea of structure can be helpful to organise your consultation, although, as we shall see, it's important to be able to work with this structure quite flexibly at times.

There's a lot of very useful material out there on the ideal model for structuring consultations. In fact it was one of the earliest topics of research on contemporary healthcare communication, with Byrne and Long's (1976) study of a 'typical' primary care interview.[6] More recent work, such as Roger Neighbour's *The Inner Consultation* (2005)[3] and the Calgary–Cambridge team (2005),[2] have built on this in setting out roughly similar models for the ideal structure and progression for a GP consultation. In all of these works the phases of the consultation follow the order outlined in Table 4.2 above.

In our data from the CSA, we mapped 40 consultations, high scoring and low scoring, to see what kind of structure they followed. The majority of candidates, high scoring and lower scoring, all stuck to the rough structure, outlined above, during **routine cases**. They did however adapt this slightly during more **complex cases**.

'Routine cases' were all those cases that required a relatively straightforward clinical diagnosis, from information discussed during data-gathering. The majority of the cases in the CSA do fall into this routine category, so it's important to look at how they work. If we look at the time spent on these six phases as a graph, we can see what most of the routine cases look like (Figure 4.1).

The structure of these routine consultations looks a bit like 'half-time' at a match. The data-gathering begins quickly after the first few opening lines and takes up roughly the

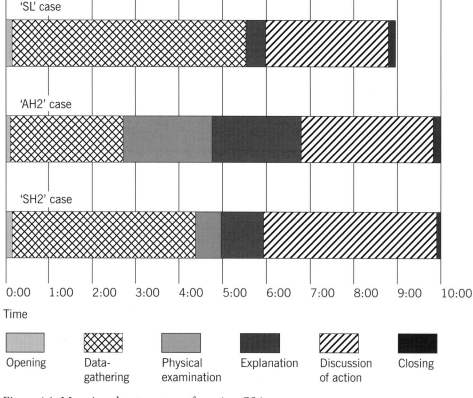

*Figure 4.1* Mapping the structure of routine CSA cases

next 3:00–4:30 minutes of the consultation. Certainly by just after the 'half-time' 5:00 minute marker, most candidates are switching the direction of the talk. They're wrapping up the data-gathering and getting into a medical explanation and clinical management plan with the patient.

The majority of candidates know this 'half-time' structure well, which is hardly surprising given years of medical training. You've probably used this structure thousands of times. Nevertheless it's useful to know that it generally works for routine cases in the exam as well. You can also see a few things that go wrong. …

### Structuring – late data-gathering

There was one pattern associated with lower-scoring candidates – where a data-gathering phase occurred well after 'half-time'. It tended to be associated with lower marks. This could occur for all sorts of reasons – a candidate forgetting to ask an important question, or a new piece of information coming to light during the management discussion that then had to be explored. For example, in this discussion of a female patient's genital herpes, they discuss, just before the 'half-time' marker, that it was likely to have been contracted from her husband. The candidate has begun his explanation then:

*Mrs D – extract 1 – 4:00 minutes into the consultation*

```
RPL:    but how did I get it
CAN:    um in the first place
RPL:    yeah
CAN:    it's normally a a sexually transmitted infection
(pause)
RPL:    oh (pause) ok (pause)
        so that means that I got it from my husband then
(pause)
CAN:    um you've how long have you been married for
RPL:    six years
CAN:    so there there is a small chance you could have had it
        before and this is the first time it's shown up (pause) um or
RPL:    what so it can take that long
(pause)
RPL:    so I could have had it all this time and it just didn't (pause) sort of
CAN:    po- potentially
RPL:    show itself or whatever
CAN:    that that is one possibility (.)
        um or as you say you may have
(pause)
RPL:    is that a likely possibility
CAN:    um (pause) it's for a slight possibility to be honest with you
RPL:    a slight possibility
CAN:    mmm
(pause)
RPL:    the chances are it's more likely to have happened in the last six
        years (.) is that what you're saying
CAN:    I am saying that yeah I'm sorry
(pause)
RPL:    ok (pause) um
(pause)
CAN:    sorry I know it's a very difficult situation
(pause)
RPL:    so that means he's been cheating basically
(pause)
RPL:    is that (.) pretty much the crux of it
CAN:    I ob- obviously I couldn't say one hundred percent
        do you think you'll be able to talk to your husband
RPL:    yeah I guess I'll have to (pause)
RPL:    I'll kill him
```

The poor fictional husband so far seems likely to take the brunt of the blame for this diagnosis. However, it transpires later, nearly 8 minutes into this consultation, that the patient's husband has a cold sore and this may be a more likely cause. The candidate has to back-track and conduct some new data-gathering, exploring the new possibility that this has not been contracted because of the husband's infidelity:

*Mrs D – extract 2 – 7:50 minutes into the consultation*

```
RPL:    cos I haven't been having sex with anyone else
```

```
CAN:    mmm
RPL:    so
CAN:    it's (.) it it's it's most likely so
RPL:    I mean
(pause)
CAN:    would do you want to
RPL:    cos you said it was like a cold sore virus I don't don't see what
        cold sores have anything to do with it
CAN:    ok um
        it's because it's the same sort of virus well there's two
        different types the one you get from (.)
        sort of direct contact (.)
        er like kissing and things like that
RPL:    cos he's got a cold sore
CAN:    ok (.) um
(pause)
CAN:    ok and (.) when you have sex with (.)
        does is he um do you ever do cunnilingus like oral sex
(pause)
RPL:    yeah
CAN:    ok
```

This kind of situation, especially important information coming to light quite late in the 10-minute case, is probably every candidate's exam nightmare. The candidate above certainly struggled to get back on track. Protracted misunderstandings like this did form part of poorer-performing candidates' exams. It's certainly not ideal, but anybody can make a mistake and there were some strategies candidates used to do this 'late' data-gathering as well as possible. It could certainly be done in a way that still meant candidates succeeded with managing the case correctly, just as it can in real-life situations where something has been forgotten.

Deciding when to ask your forgotten question is important. The following candidate, who encounters a number of problems, has a problem early on with a forgotten question. While he's giving an explanation on his diagnostic decision, he cuts the explanation short. He quickly interjects his forgotten question:

*Mrs H – extract 1*

```
CAN:    and and your examination is fine
RPL:    right good good
CAN:    er a problem you are describing I mean it is fairly common
RPL:    right yes
CAN:    er it is called menorrhagia
RPL:    right
CAN:    wh- which means that er erm er
        women do hav- do bleed quite heavily
        er one thing which I forgot to ask
        I mean is it painful when when
RPL:    er no
CAN:    alright er so yeah I mean er your smear was fine a few weeks er er a
        few months ago hh- er there isn't any other sign which would worry me
```

```
RPL:    right
CAN:    now there are a couple of options that we can use. …
```

It's not a complicated question that he's missed. However, a few things go wrong that cause confusion. Explanation sequences are quite important and, as we'll see below, when you begin to describe a medical term like this …

```
CAN:    er it is called menorrhagia wh- which means that er erm er women do
        hav- do bleed quite heavily
```

… it tends to signal the start of a relatively lengthy explanation phase, where the candidate will talk for a while. It's a kind of **mini-explanation** structure, and often used as an opening to explanation phases. Cutting this phase very short means that he has only given a minimal explanation of his diagnostic decision, which the role-player doesn't have a chance to respond to. After his question, the candidate goes straight back into describing the diagnostic decision, albeit with a little bit of trouble: 'alright er so yeah I mean er …', immediately followed by treatment options. Placing forgotten questions after an explanation sequence has been completed, even if not entirely smooth, can still work better for you than quickly interjecting them as soon as you think of them. It gives the role-player a chance to respond to the explanation (we'll talk more about openings in Chapter 5).

Similarly, this candidate also has to ask a forgotten question 6 minutes into his case. Overall, he did very well in the CSA, so anyone can make mistakes like these. The next example is from a case about a woman, Mrs T, who has come to the doctor to discuss her incontinence. The candidate has established during the consultation that her problem is likely to be stress incontinence and has discussed the option of seeing a physiotherapist.

*Mrs T case – extract 1*

```
CAN:    so you need to continue them
        for six weeks to see how well they've worked
RPL:    and this is something that will help stop
CAN:    it (.) should help
        whether it stops the problem or not
        is difficult to say until we've done the exercises
        y- know if the exercises haven't worked
        then we can try an-
        try a try the medication
RPL:    ok
```

However, he realises he has forgotten an important question in taking a full history for stress incontinence.

```
CAN:    ok (.) um the other thing I I spec- I forgot to ask you earlier on was
        do ever get a sensation of something coming down down below um
        (0.8)
RPL:    no
CAN:    ok right oh
        um (.) sometimes (.) um you can (.)
        the neck of the womb can kind of come down as well
        and it it probably be a good idea for us to
        have a look to make sure that wasn't there
```

```
        (1.3)
CAN:    would you be ok if I did that with a nurse or would you
RPL:    yeah I mean could you tell me what you're going to do
CAN:    ok basically want to look at the neck of the womb
        to see whether it's it's coming down as well
        especially I'll I'll be getting you to cough so if you cough
        and the neck of the womb comes down um there's other treatments that
        we could offer … it would be a speculum examination
```

Unlike the candidate in the previous case we looked at (Mrs H), this candidate waits until he has finished giving his explanation of the treatment options before then asking the question. Some of the false starts and hesitations in this section might indicate a bit of trouble here for the candidate, and it can be difficult to make these forgotten questions look completely smooth. However, his hesitation doesn't matter too much because, overall, he manages to get this section done well and importantly he gets the work done in a way that the patient aligns with. More importantly still, he is then able successfully to go back and cover this important part of the data-gathering, describing a speculum examination for which he then receives the results. He passes the case.

Waiting until a relevant point to make this topic transition to the forgotten question, rather than quickly interjecting it in an explanation as the first candidate did, means that the consultation flows more easily. It also means that the candidate has space to then properly ask about carrying out an additional physical examination – one that he needed to do as part of his data-gathering to pass the case. Although late data-gathering causes some real difficulties with the structure and the alignment created with the patient, there are strategies for adding in missing sections of data-gathering or forgotten questions that can help to get these done in the clearest way possible – so, if this happens, don't panic and find a suitable place to ask your forgotten question.

### Flexible structure in complex cases

We've looked at some structuring in routine cases, consisting of a relatively straightforward sequence of data-gathering, diagnosis and treatment discussion with the role-played patient, and how to manage things if that typical structure goes off-track with some late data-gathering. However, we've also said that candidates had to deviate from this in more complex cases, which we'll look at now.

A 'complex' case refers not to the difficulty of the clinical problem but to the complexity of the interaction. They are often the cases where the role-played patient adopts a stance that it is very difficult for the GP to fully support. This complexity is most obvious in ethically oriented cases, where the views of the patient conflict with the doctor and his or her professional position. However, even though doctor and patient cannot fully agree, there can be a level of mutual respect and understanding, '**alignment**', in how the discussion proceeds. For example, this is the initial request by a role-player, Mrs C, who has come to see the doctor about her son:

*Mrs C case – extract 1*

```
RPL:    i've come about my son John
CAN:    alright
```

```
RPL:    i'd be very grateful if you could er (0.2) change his medication from
        tablets (0.7) into ones that dissolve
```

She quickly follows this initial request with a hint towards the crux of the case:

```
RPL:    so (.) I decided the only thing to do was for me to (1.7) well (0.5)
        for me to intercede and I would (0.7) breaking up these tablets which
        is quite hard to do hhhh erm (0.3) and sprinkling them on his (.)
        breakfast (.) cereal
```

Similarly, the Mr J case, which we'll look at in Chapter 5, involves a role-player who has asked for a vasectomy, but would like to keep it secret from his partner.

Rather than provide an explanation of the medication or what a vasectomy involves, these types of cases involve the candidate correctly **making inferences** about the moral problem at stake. Such cases often don't have a straightforward resolution or even require a final decision within the 10 minutes. There is not necessarily a 'right' answer, but the candidate is expected to show a mode of approach that is justifiable. They usually require identifying the problem and discussing sensitively so that the interaction does not break down in conflict. So rather than the 'half-time' switchover we saw above, these cases can have a whole range of structures, leaving room for what we've called a 'Key Problem Discussion' between the role-player and the candidate. They look quite different (see Figure 4.2).

We used the label 'Key Problem Discussion' to describe a quite different kind of task, where the role-player and GP both need the space to talk about their respective stances. For example, in the Mr J case, which we'll see examples from in Chapter 5, the candidate has to conduct a much slower discussion of the issue at stake. The patient has asked for

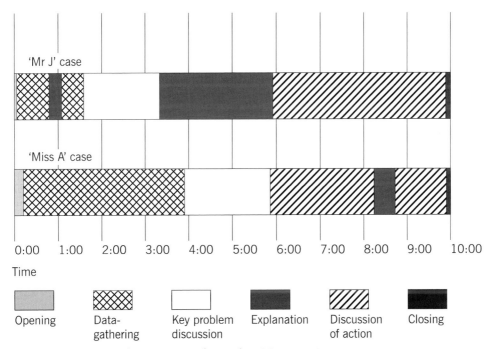

*Figure 4.2* Mapping the structure of complex CSA cases

a vasectomy referral, but wants to know if this can be done secretly, without his partner finding out. The doctor is going to have to manage a tricky ethical discussion with a patient whose position she might not agree with. Her role as a GP means she cannot be judgemental about the patient's request or insist that he disclose confidential medical information to his partner, but she is also obliged to discuss the effect that his request might have on significant others. So the work of the consultation means balancing the discussion of medical aspects of having a vasectomy with the ethical discussion of the potential impact on his life and those around him.

So the important idea to take from this is that there will be occasions when you need to be a bit flexible with the structure. It's useful for any of the consultations to figure out what kind of case you're dealing with and to think about where you might need to take the consultation, but it's especially important for these more ethically oriented cases, where you'll need a bit of space for discussion. We'll talk a bit about ideas for how to make these '**inferences**' early on in the consultation.

### Top tips – structuring

The three-part structure of data-gathering – explanation – clinical management, switching roughly around or just after 'half-time', is a model that works well for most routine cases in the exam.

Be careful to think through your data-gathering and try to ask all the questions you need to make a diagnosis before that magic 'half-time' changeover.

However, if you do make a mistake and forget something, don't panic, because there are ways to get your consultation back on track and do well. Think about where the best place to ask your forgotten question will be – don't do it right in the middle of giving a medical explanation, but finish off your topic and then flag up your new topic change (for example 'Another thing I'd like to ask is …'). This gives you the space to think through and structure a new set of questions without confusing your role-played patient – or even, as one candidate here did, conduct a second physical examination and still manage the case correctly.

Some cases are going to require more flexibility with the structure, particularly those ethics-based or tricky cases where the role-played patient adopts a stance that the GP can't fully **align** with. For example, we briefly looked at the Mrs C case (see pp. 32–3), where the mother would like to administer medication to her son without his knowledge, and in Chapter 5 we will look at the Mr J case (see pp. 38–9) where a man would like a secret vasectomy. There are also some more complex cases in the practice role-plays for this book, such as the assisted dying case. In terms of the structuring, these more complex cases often required the candidate to leave room for a much slower 'Key Problem Discussion' phase, where both parties, GP and player, have space to talk about their positions and the difficulties of the situation.

*Exercise – Structuring*

Take one of the more routine cases from the practice exam cases in Part II and have a go at performing it with two other colleagues. One of you can play the candidate, one the role-played patient and the third the examiner. Read through the paperwork that has been provided, for the candidate, the examiner and the role-player, and try out a 10-minute test-run of the case, with the 'examiner' keeping a strict start–stop time. The 'examiner' can try to listen out for the features listed on the mark sheet, but importantly, for this exercise, he or she should also roughly mark when the three general tasks data-gathering, diagnosis or explanation and discussion of action all occur. There might be more than one phase where these occur of course. How long does the GP spend on each of these tasks? Did the typical three-part structure work well in managing the case? After this, try swapping roles and timing each of the sections again – although of course the later 'candidates' will have a great advantage in planning out the structure, having seen the case already!

## References

1. Roberts C, Atkins S, Hawthorne K. *Performance Features in Clinical Skills Assessment: Linguistic and Cultural Factors in the Membership of the Royal College of General Practitioners Examination.* London: King's College London and Centre for Language Discourse and Communication, 2014, www.kcl.ac.uk/sspp/departments/education/research/ldc/publications/MRCGPling/MRCGPling.aspx [accessed 10 April 2015].
2. Kurtz S, Silverman J, Draper J. *Teaching and Learning Communication Skills in Medicine.* 2nd edn. Abingdon: Radcliffe Publishing, 2005.
3. Neighbour R. *The Inner Consultation: How to Develop an Effective and Intuitive Consulting Style.* 2nd edn. Abingdon: Radcliffe Publishing, 2005.
4. The Consultation Observation Tool. www.rcgp.org.uk/gp-training-and-exams/mrcgp-workplace-based-assessment-wpba/cot-for-mrcgp-workplace-based-assessment.aspx [accessed 22 January 2015].
5. RCGP Online Learning Environment. Clinical Skills Assessment. http://elearning.rcgp.org.uk/csa [accessed 2 June 2015].
6. Byrne PS, Long BE. *Doctors Talking to Patients.* London: HMSO, 1976.
7. Heritage J, Maynard D. *Communication in Medical Care: Interaction between Primary Care Physicians and Patients.* Cambridge: Cambridge University Press, 2006.

# 5   Looking closely at talk in different phases of the consultation

*Sarah Atkins and Celia Roberts*

In Chapter 4, we introduced some general ideas about the communicative requirements of the Clinical Skills Assessment (CSA), particularly how entire cases are structured by candidates, and features that characterised good performance. We broke that structure down into a series of tasks, including data-gathering, physical examination, explanation and discussion of action. We'll now look in more detail at how this series of tasks, which we've addressed quite abstractly in the sequence of the case, is actually achieved. After all, it's the details of how talk is done that can be the most helpful in picking up hints and tips to use in your consultations.

## Getting started and data-gathering

We talked a bit about the importance of figuring out the direction the case is likely to go in, so that you can start working out a structure for the talk early on, particularly for complex cases. Let's start by looking at the openings of cases and the inferences and conversational moves that the GP and role-player make early in the consultation during data-gathering.

### Opening lines and scripts

Roger Neighbour (2005) talks about the importance of the opening few seconds of a consultation in his book *The Inner Consultation*.[1] He calls these 'gambits and curtain-raisers':

> In chess, some of the opening moves are called 'gambits'. One player makes a move calculated to draw a particular response from the opponent, which the gambit-maker hopes can be turned to his own advantage. Patients make opening gambits too. The first thing a patient says is the only part of the consultation he or she has much control over. … While patients are waiting their turn to see you, they are usually silently rehearsing exactly what it is they are planning to say, how they are going to begin, how they are going to explain their symptoms or their requests.[1]

Neighbour suggests a great deal can be gleaned from the patient's slightly rehearsed opening gambit then, on what the consultation will likely be about. In particular, he addresses the idea that certain comments, 'curtain raisers', help reveal a lot about the way the patient perceives you and how the consultation is going to go.

Roberts *et al.* (2004) identify how, in real life, eliciting a patient's symptoms, feelings, ideas and expectations in these opening few lines does not always run in the orderly way communication models might imply.[2] In their data from GP consultations in Lambeth, a borough of London, patients who shared the same cultural and linguistic resources as the GP did indeed give these fairly long opening preambles and frame their own stance to their symptoms. However, patients with other cultural backgrounds, who had perhaps not been socialised in this particular model of the GP consultation, could manage this presentation in different ways, sometimes disrupting the GP's expected model for the interaction. Roberts *et al.* highlight, therefore, the wide variety of expectations that patients bring to the consultation and the different manner in which they express this in the opening few lines.

Cases in the CSA do have an important 'opening line' from the role-played patient, but it looks rather different from any of the models or studies of 'real-life' talk. While there's no patient sat in the waiting room rehearsing, as there is in Neighbour's Inner Consultation model, the role-player has been rehearsing his or her role beforehand and most likely performing it repeatedly between candidates. So their opening gambit will be a well-polished, rehearsed couple of lines, usually quite a bit shorter than you see in 'real' consultations. For example:

### *Opening lines*

#### *Opening lines – Mrs D – extract 3*

```
CAN:    hi it's Mrs D
RPL:    hi yeah
CAN:    hi I'm doctor ****** please come and take a seat
RPL:    hello
(pause)
CAN:    hi (.) what can I do for you today
RPL:    um (.) about three weeks ago (.) I got (.) had these spots down below
CAN:    mmhmm
RPL:    um but they're cleared now
(pause)
CAN:    (nods) ok and
(pause)
CAN:    do you want to tell me a bit more about it …
```

#### *Opening lines – Mr R – extract 1*

```
CAN:    come in (0.4) Mr R**** (.) hello I'm doctor ****
RPL:    hi
CAN:    please have a seat
(pause)
CAN:    yes
(pause)
RPL:    er it's er::: a bit embarrassing doctor
CAN:    mhm
```

```
RPL:     I've got a problem with my sex life
(pause)
CAN:     ok
RPL:     yeah
(pause)
CAN:     do you want to tell me a bit more about it
```

Many candidates had this exact same way of responding to this opening gambit:

```
'do you want to tell me a bit more about …'
```

In fact, statistically, this phrase occurs far more frequently in the CSA than in any other setting – it's much more frequent than everyday talk and much more frequent than in regular, day-to-day GP surgeries. This makes it an 'exam phrase', or what we shall call '**formulaic phrases**' – phrases and words that occur together very frequently. This finding came out of conducting a quantitative analysis of the CSA transcripts, which you can read more about in Roberts et al.[2] The method used to identify these phrases takes all the transcribed CSA cases we made as a dataset and compared this with other, larger reference datasets to see what comes up more or less frequently. Other phrases that came up frequently later in the opening to CSA cases were variations of:

```
'What were you hoping I could do for you today …'
'What do you think is going on …'
'What do you think might be causing this …'
```

You can see why these kind of phrases occur so often. It's a good way to give the role-played patient the chance to speak very freely about what he or she thinks is important to the consultation and what he or she expects, just as the Calgary–Cambridge model suggests:

> An excellent way to explore the patient's perspective and some of the issues involved in eliciting it is to look at the phrasing of direct questions that ask patients for their ideas and concerns. Bring out the difficulties of phrasing such questions so that both doctor and patient feel comfortable. … *Produce separate lists* of possible phrases for ideas and concerns. … *Practising exact phrases* can be very helpful (e.g. *'What were you hoping for today?'*)[3]

These kind of phrases can be useful of course – they give you something pre-rehearsed to use in a consultation or a stressful exam. There's nothing wrong with them. All professional fields and indeed exams have characteristic phrases and ways of talking that are used to perform required tasks. But you also need to be careful that not everything you say is just from a pre-prepared script. Many of the candidates' videos we analysed in our study were found, by examiners, at times to sound too formulaic. Sometimes, it might not be that appropriate to ask the patient 'do you want to tell me a bit more about …'. Not all candidates had to use these pre-rehearsed phrases to do very well. For example, the candidate who does well in the Mr J case, starts in this way:

*Opening lines – Mr J – extract 1*

```
CAN:     hello hi there come in
```

```
RPL:    hi doctor hi thank you
CAN:    mr j*****
RPL:    yeah that's right yes
(pause)
CAN:    my name is dr ***** how can I help you this morning
RPL:    um I'd like a referral for a vasectomy please
CAN:    right (.) ok um you must have been thinking about that for **** ****
ok
RPL:    yeah I suppose so yes yes yes
CAN:    tell me a little bit about your thoughts about it
```

So, while formulaic phases can be useful much of the time, you don't have to use them every time and particularly not at moments where they feel inappropriate.

### Getting started and making inferences in complex cases

In the section on structuring in the previous chapter, we saw a case where the patient requests a vasectomy that he wants to keep secret from his partner. We'll explore the complex requirements of this case in a little more depth. The candidate does well in the case, avoiding overt disagreements and managing the discussion well. Part of her success is in how she sets up this balancing act right at the start. Look at how she continues:

*Mr J – extract 2*

```
CAN:    I do have a few details in your records
        I notice that you're not currently in a relationship
RPL:    oh I am yes yes yes yes
CAN:    oh you are ok can you tell me a bit about that
RPL:    oh well I mean we've been together for a long time I mean yeah I mean
        I I
CAN:    mmhmm
RPL:    seldom need to come in here so I don't know how old the records are
        but er
CAN:    oh they must be quite old
RPL:    er b- yeah I mean we've we've lived together for years so
CAN:    right
RPL:    yeah
CAN:    ok and is this um is this a decision that you've taken together
        is it something that
RPL:    um I'd probably say it's my decision
CAN:    ok
RPL:    ummm last time we chatted about things was a few years ago
CAN:    ok
RPL:    and I know that we didn't want any children then and I know that
CAN:    yeah yes
RPL:    I don't want any children now so so I feel as though you know
CAN:    yeah
RPL:    it's my decision to make
CAN:    ok is your partner female male
RPL:    yes female yeah
CAN:    if you mind me asking ok and is there something
```

```
                  now er er I know you've just said it's your decision to make
RPL:     mmm
CAN:     and I completely agree
RPL:     mmm
CAN:     is it something that she's aware that you've been thinking about
         is it something that you've talked about (.) together
RPL:     er no
CAN:     right
RPL:     no I mean it's you know I I I feel as though
         I'd I'd (.) prefer to do it to do it myself er
CAN:     ok
RPL:     yeah
CAN:     do you mind me asking for what reason
RPL:     um I I have a slight inkling that she might be a bit little bit broody
         at the moment
CAN:     right
RPL:     um and um I know that I (.) don't want to make her pregnant
CAN:     ok
RPL:     um (.) so I feel as though (.) this is
RPL:     my choice to make I suppose
CAN:     ok
RPL:     yeah
CAN:     have you considered any other options that might be available to you
```

Her early questioning strategy is designed to get longer responses from the role-player so that she can understand the reasons for his request, although she adapts the frequently used questions we saw such as, 'can you tell me a little bit more about it …' quite a lot:

```
'you must have been thinking about that'
'tell me a little bit about your thoughts about it'
```

Much like the first candidate we looked at in the Mr O case above, she first asks about his prior medical understanding of what a vasectomy involves:

```
CAN:     tell me a little bit about what you know about vasectomy already, um,
         have you done any reading or have you spoken to anybody about it
```

She 'signposts' (see pp. 46–7 for an exploration of 'signposting') that she'll go into the medical aspects of vasectomy in a little more detail later, but before she does this she also asks about his partner:

```
CAN:     I do have a few details in your records I notice that you're not
         currently in a relationship
RPL:     oh I am yes yes yes yes
CAN:     oh you are ok can you tell me a bit about that
         […]
CAN:     ok and is this um is this a decision that you've taken together is it
         something that
```

Her data-gathering is therefore a balance of asking medically oriented questions about his understanding of vasectomy, but also these more socially and perhaps morally oriented questions about his life circumstances. She's able to make some inferences, early on then, about the type of case this is. **Making inferences** is a tricky but very useful skill in tackling more complex cases. As Neighbour notes, the opening 'curtain raisers' from the patient can tell you a lot about where the case might go.[1] The same is true in the CSA role-plays. In particular, you can often start recognising, early on, those cases where there might be more complex issues to tackle. Spotting these complex cases early on will obviously help you grapple with how to structure the consultation. We saw earlier how complex cases in particular could require some flexibility with structure, so figuring this out early on is clearly going to help plan for that. Of course, your initial inferences might not always turn out to be quite right, so be prepared to listen out for more cues as the data-gathering goes on.

There's sometimes a danger of reading too much into what a patient says or how he or she says it, which can lead to a few hiccups. This candidate, in a case with a young woman who has attended the GP about an unplanned pregnancy, makes an inference about what the patient has said about her concerns with talking to her partner:

```
CAN:    … but I know you were also worried that he may pressurise you into into
        keeping it when it you feel it's not the right time
(pause)
RPL:    I don't know that I f- I jus- I don't I don't that was my concern um
        um I don't
(pause)
RPL:    yeah
CAN:    what's what what else is troubling you
        I mean obviously this is a serious situation was there anything else
        that was bothering you at all
(pause)
RPL:    I just don't know how the hell I'm going to make a choice like
        this I don't know where to start or (.) or what's going to make me
        decide li- i just have no idea what to do
CAN:    ok alright hhh um (.) and I guess you came today for for advice and um
        answers really
```

The inference was clearly not quite right and they must do a little repair work to establish that there is nothing in particular about her relationship that is worrying her, but that she has attended to ask for advice on her unplanned pregnancy. Overall, though, they manage to repair this short misunderstanding well and the candidate does well in the case.

It is a difficult line to tread between picking up on everything the role-played patient is indicating and jumping to too many conclusions. Nevertheless, while it's important to be careful about making inferences and not jump to hasty conclusions or sweeping generalisations, overall it's a very useful technique in the exam, even if you make a few slip-ups on the way. Making inferences was a frequent feature of successful candidates in the CSA and it begins right from these opening few lines from the role-player.

---

### Exercise – Making inferences in complex cases

After you've had a go at the practice cases in Chapters 7 and 8, go back and look at the opening gambit that was written in the case notes for the role-player. Were there any signs as to the direction the case might go in? What were the first inferences that popped into your head and were any of them right? Note down what the patient said next in your role-play and see if there were any other indicators you could have picked up on.

*Table 5.1* Mr O's blood pressure results card

|  | *Blood pressure* | *Pulse* |
|---|---|---|
| 2 weeks ago | 165/100, 162/94, 158/90 | 72 |
| 1 week ago | 160/95, 158/96, 162/92 | 70 |
| Today | 158/96, 162/92, 164/94 | 74 |
| ECG | Mild LVH only |  |

### Structuring questions

We've seen how candidates conduct the opening few lines of a CSA consultation with what have classically been called 'open questions', which allow the patient an open space to describe his or her concerns. But let's also look a little more closely at other types of questioning strategy. Communication skills textbooks often talk about open-ended questions and, indeed, they're very useful for getting long responses out of the role-player or patient. However, there's a time and a place for quick questions and they can be very useful in an exam, especially when you need to get a lot of work done quickly. Data-gathering in the 10-minute CSA consultation can become a fine balance of all sorts of different question types.

In this case, Mr O, the role-player, has come to find out about some test results. The role-player portrays a patient who has been referred to the GP by the practice nurse for his high blood pressure. The GP has notes in front of her indicating Mr O has been sent in by the practice nurse. She's had a couple of minutes to read these before the whistle sounds and Mr O comes through the door carrying the results of his blood pressure tests.

*Example – Mr O opening*

```
CAN:    come in hello there hi mister O my name is doctor *****
RPL:    hello
CAN:    sorry you are *******
RPL:    I am yes yes
CAN:    yeah just checking ok
        how can I help you sir today
RPL:    um well I was I asked to see by the
        nurse about blo- blood pressure she's just tested it again
CAN:    ok
RPL:    so it's
CAN:    right let's have a look (pause) so
(pause)
CAN:    right so today um it's a little bit high it seems and ok
RPL:    right
CAN:    it were you aware of that or
RPL:    no
CAN:    did she say anything to you at all
RPL:    no
CAN:    no ok so you're not quite sure why the nurse sent you in isn't that
        ok
RPL:    no well er what you just said to
```

```
CAN:    right ok now um it sounds like she's done three blood pressure
        readings all sort of
RPL:    that's right yeah
(pause)
CAN:    er a week apart really
RPL:    uh-huh …
```

(You can see the clip for this in the RCGP's e-learning module.)[4]

The candidate establishes a shared way of addressing the problem early on in the consultation. The first thing she does, then, is to ask the role-player, fairly open-endedly, why he's come. The role-player mentions the nurse sending him in about his blood pressure and the candidate gets into the work of the consultation, looking at his test results card. **'right let's have a look (.) so…'** is a very collaborative way of **'signposting'** (see pp. 46–7 on signposting) that they are going to go through the test results together – it won't just be her looking through them. It also sounds conversational and gives her a pause to read the card. Starting off in this way gives the candidate and role-player a collaborative way of going through the test results. The measured tempo gives the candidate a chance to read the card and to go fairly slowly when she's asking the role-player about his understanding.

She gives the news that his blood pressure is 'a little bit high', followed by a short explanation on what the blood pressure tests were for. What the candidate is good at doing throughout her consultation is giving **'information sandwiches'**, something she starts doing from this early stage in the consultation. She gives her signpost, followed by a bit of information and then checks the role-player's prior understanding about his tests. For the candidate this is a useful way to gather information about what the patient already knows.

```
CAN:    right let's have a look (.) so …                       signpost
        (pause)
        right so today um it's a little bit high it seems and  information
        ok
RPL:    right
CAN:    it were you aware of that or ↘                          checking
RPL:    no
CAN:    did she say anything to you at all                      checking
RPL:    no
CAN:    no ok
CAN:    so you're not quite sure why the nurse sent you in isn't  checking
        that (.) ok
RPL:    no well er what you just said to
```

These answers from the role-player are fairly short, compared with the longer, more open-ended replies we saw with Mr J above. Nevertheless, the candidate takes the 'checking understanding' questions quite slowly, allowing him more space to reply should he want to.

Straight after this introduction of the topic, she uses the same sandwich technique again.

```
CAN:   right ok now um it sounds like                    signpost
       she's done three blood pressure readings all sort of    information
RPL:   that's right yeah (pause)
CAN:   er a week apart really                            information
RPL:   uh-huh
CAN:   and what we look at is the bottom and the top value    information
       now is er have you ever had your blood pressure
       checked before
RPL:   mm no
CAN:   do you know much about blood pressure ⌍            checking
RPL:   er j- just what it roughly does look you know heart
       and the breathing and all that keeps going
CAN:   yeah yeah the reason we check is
```

The relatively slow pace, and particularly the shift when she switches to questions that check Mr O's knowledge, gives the role-player the chance to make a slightly lengthier response. Once again she also changes her pitch downwards when she switches to the checking questions, signalling the shift from giving information to something a bit more personal.

If you're able to watch the video on the RCGP e-learning site, you can also take a look at how good she is at sharing the card of blood test results, in a way that Mr O can see it and the figures she's pointing to (which can feel tricky to do in an exam setting where you're sat across from the patient with an overseeing examiner). She then looks up from the card to check his prior understanding about blood pressure.

This structure of signpost – information – checking is one method you can try, but you might have your own ways of delivering information, in a way that attends to the relationship with the patient and his or her understanding. Have a look at the ways you do this, either in role-plays or, if you can, from videos of your own consultations and see if you can tease out the other kinds of strategies you use that might be useful.

After this slightly slower, initial checking phase, about a minute and a half into the consultation, she then gets into some more targeted data-gathering.

*Example – Mr O*

```
line
49 RPL: right yeah
50 CAN: but can I just ask you sp- some specific questions about it if that's
        ok
51 RPL: of course yeah
52 CAN: now um have you noticed sort of any headaches recently
53 RPL: no
54 CAN: no any problems with your vision at all
55 RPL: no
56 CAN: not feels not felt sick or unwell
57 RPL: no
58 CAN: no ok and (pause) prior to this visit I mean what what was the reason
59      why you sorry went to the practice nurse in the first place
```

```
60 RPL:        oh it was it's my wife's command
61 CAN: oh as yeah ok
62 RPL: but no she is er I was fifty last week and er sort of couple weeks back
63      she said you know we're hitting big one you may as well have an M-O-T
        so
64 CAN: yeah I kind of thought way er sorry for me just to assume that really
        ok fine
```

You might notice in the video available through the RCGP e-learning for this excerpt that the candidate speeds up a little to go through these questions. The role-player, recognising the change of pace, gives short, one-word answers. You can see his short, one-word 'no' responses.

This **quick questioning** strategy is absolutely fine for many parts of data-gathering. It can often be very useful, once you have established a more open start to the consultation, to then ask some very structured medical history questions, and for many medical conditions you will probably have practised a particular sequence of important and structured history questions many times with patients in your clinic. The important thing is that the patient aligns with this questioning and the GP is also flexible in slowing the pace down again when needed.

Being able to switch between speeds is an important skill. She has started very collaboratively, but now speeds up into what might be thought of as a more 'doctor-centred' style. The role-player does not have the same opportunity here to give the longer, conversational responses that he did in the first minute. Some research suggests many patients understand and align with these quick questions quite well in GP consultations. Certainly you can see here, in this routine case, that the role-player gets on board with the change of pace and the quick questions go smoothly. The talk is **aligned** (see p. 26) in the sense that both speakers are in agreement about the work they are doing.

---

### Exercise – 'Quick questions'

*Part 1*

Using the results card that Mr O brings in have a go at delivering the information on the blood pressure test results. You could also plan for the questions you want to ask Mr O over the course of data-gathering – and which questions you might want to ask in a **quick question** structure. You could practise this as a role-play with a group of trainees. Given the average time spent on this phase, you want to plan to talk for about 4–5 minutes in this exercise, which can feel pretty short when you're under pressure! But that's why it's useful to practise under exam conditions.

*Part 2*

Take a look at the Mr O extract above and see if you can identify what she does before she starts this questioning sequence. What might you term the move she makes at line 50 before moving into the 'quick questions'?

```
'can I just ask you sp- some specific questions about it if that's ok'
```

Why is this an important part of the whole question sequence?

---

### Exercise – Part 2 discussion

Linguists and communication skills textbooks have variously described what this candidate does in line 50:

```
'can I just ask you sp- some specific questions about it if that's ok'
```

It can be called 'asking permission' before going on to a detailed set of questions, a strategy often used in the CSA, especially when asking more personal questions. Asking permission is part of showing your awareness and concern for the role-played patient, indicating that he or she has some level of choice in how the interaction goes. Here the candidate waits for the role-player's answer: 'of course yeah', before moving on to asking the rapid set of questions we just saw.

This kind of strategy can also be called 'signposting', flagging up what's coming up next in the talk. It's often discussed in communication skills models and is a hugely important feature of GP and CSA talk. We're going to talk about 'signposting' a lot more in the next section.

---

## Key concept: Signposting and 'metacommunication'

Metacommunication is a useful term from linguistics, which we want to introduce in this section. We'll come back to it throughout the chapter and it's a big part of the e-learning module we mentioned. Metacommunication is all the talk you do *about* your talk, a kind of commentary you can give that helps the listener interpret what you're saying. Very often, the giveaway that we're metacommunicating is that there will be some kind of description specifically about talk:

```
'If we talk a bit about you know …'
'can I just ask you sp- some specific questions …'
'It's a funny term cystic fibrosis …'
```

We do this all the time when we're talking, even in casual conversation, giving a kind of online commentary as we're speaking. It's really useful to think about how you do this in the CSA.

Previously, we started thinking about a simple but very useful way of metacommunicating – 'signposting'. You have probably encountered this idea of signposting before – letting the patient know where the consultation is going and what's coming next. It's a very clear strategy candidates use to make what comes next more expected for the role-player or patient.

```
'right let's have a look (.) so …'
'can I just ask you some specific questions …'
```

It's understandably a very oft-cited strategy in communication skills textbooks. Lloyd and Bor's (2009) *Communication Skills for Medicine* recommends:

> Signposts on a road direct us toward our destination and keep us on the right track. In the same way, signposting during a consultation indicates to the patient what you

want to discuss next and is a valuable part of effective communication. Examples of signposting are: '*And now I want to ask you a few more questions about…*'.[5]

Signposting is certainly a very useful feature in consultations and it's very frequent in the CSA. The candidate's use of signposting in the case of Mr O, before asking some '**quick questions**', is certainly a very important way of making sure the talk is aligned and the patient is happy to answer some targeted history taking. We can see it's successful because the patient gets on board and aligns with the talk by giving some short yes/ no answers. Successful candidates use these kinds of signposts throughout their consultations in the CSA and they can point to things that are much 'further away' in the talk. So, for example, in the Mr J case, the candidate says:

```
CAN:    it's a very effective procedure but it's
        something with quite permanent consequences
RPL:    mmm mmm
CAN:    which is something that we will go over
```

By indicating 'which is something that we will go over', this GP is pointing ahead to something that will come up in the consultation later on. It might sound like an obvious thing to say, but do make sure you return to topics that you signpost – a feature of poor-performing candidates that examiners picked up on in the research was signposted topics that were never returned to. So try to keep a mental note of your 'more distant' signposted topics.

However, you don't just have to point forwards of course; you can point backwards at something you've already said:

```
'so it can cause, which are the questions I was just asking you … it can make
you look very tanned, it can affect…'
```

The important idea to keep in mind for now is that all of these signposting strategies fall under this idea of 'metacommunication' – a kind of talk about your talk, which points to things you're going to say or have already said. You can even use it to point out specific words that are coming up:

```
'it's a funny term, cystic fibrosis, it's it's a congenital disease which
means that'
```

By saying 'it's a funny term', the candidate here flags up the particular words that might be new to the role-played patient, so signposting at a very micro-level about what's coming up in the talk and how to interpret this.

Signposting is a useful technique to help the patient understand why you're doing things, but it's an especially good idea in an exam when you also need to show the examiner you know what you're doing and where you're taking the consultation. It helps you mark out that structure we discussed above for the examiner, as well as for the role-played patient.

So that's a fairly simple way to understand 'metacommunication'. However, we can also do some much more complex things with these online, spoken commentaries than simply signpost what's coming up. But try to keep in mind, as you go through the next exercise, what some of the more complex features of metacommunication might be.

### Exercise – Signposting

One of the cases we've been looking at, Mr J, is quite complex and is worth exploring a little more in terms of the signposting she uses. (Read the opening to the case in Appendix IV.) A clip of this case is also available on the RCGP e-learning site.

The candidate does very well and she certainly uses a lot of signposting. Read through her opening couple of minutes and see if you can identify some of the signposts and how they point to tasks and talk in the consultation.

After this exercise, we'll look at more complex types of metacommunication that can be useful in conducting the consultation. So while you're reading through the case, think about any other kinds of commentary this candidate might be giving.

---

### Exercise – Signposting: discussion

There's a lot of 'signposts' in this opening section of the case. Many of them point to things the candidate is just about to say, so signposting quite close things in the talk, such as asking permission to ask a particular question:

```
line 72.
CAN: do you mind me asking for what reason
```

And to signal she is about to give some medical details:

```
lines 31-3.
CAN:    maybe I could give you a few more details
RPL:    mmm yeah yeah
CAN:    um there's a very (.) well it's a very effective procedure
```

Her signposting also points to things a bit further away, which are going to happen later in the consultation, but not in the immediate talk:

```
lines 33-6.
CAN:    um there's a very (.) well it's a very effective procedure but it's
        something with quite permanent consequences
RPL:    mmm mmm
CAN:    which is something that we will go over um
```

```
lines 99-100.
CAN:    which again I said we'll go into in just a minute so it's maybe some
        things to think about there and we'll go through that together
```

She also signposts backwards, to things the role-player has already said, demonstrating that she's received and understood what he's said and emphasising the relevance of what she says next:

```
line 29.
CAN:    ok so it sounds like you know a little bit
```

```
lines 60-3.
CAN:    I know you've just said it's your decision to make … and I completely
        agree …
```

She does many more – we've highlighted just a few here but you probably found many other examples in the exercise above. So her signposting helps you figure out how the talk is organised, at quite a local level, at the level of each speaker's turn, and also in terms of where the whole consultation is going. But we can also begin to see that it does more than this organisation and structure – we can see the useful social functions that 'metacommunication' can serve.

### Social functions of metacommunication

Subtle metacommunication goes on all the time to give a message about our particular stance and how we want our talk and identities to be interpreted. When a GP candidate adds, '... **but it's nothing for us to worry about at the moment**', after having given a short description of a symptom, she is signalling how a piece of medical information she has just given should be interpreted by the role-played patient. She's indicating that she is attentive to the relationship with the patient and their potential concerns about the content of her talk. Similarly, saying, 'It's a **funny term** cystic fibrosis' helps flag up something that might be a new term for this particular role-played patient. And we saw already it allows the GP to ask permission about where the talk is going with 'can I just **ask** you sp- some specific **questions** ...' during data-gathering, showing attentiveness to the patient. These mini-commentaries don't just signpost, then, but help to serve a social function, demonstrating a professional relationship with the addressee.

This kind of strategy can be very useful, especially in a complicated scenario like the Mr J case we looked at in the exercise and in Appendix IV. Here the candidate has to work to highlight some of the ethical difficulties with this role-played patient's request. The GP has a difficult balancing act to manage in this more ethically oriented case then. She manages to indicate her own stance to the role-player's request for a secret vasectomy – she can't fully align with his position – but she also can't be judgemental or alienate this patient entirely, so must offer some level of understanding as to the reasons for his request.

Let's look again at the last section of that transcript, lines 90–100:

```
line
90 CAN: I can see the difficulties that lie there
91      right it's a slightly unusual request I mean I see people quite often
92      asking for a vasectomies they tend to be men who are a little bit older
        who already have a family
93 RPL: mmm
94 CAN: um so it's unusual in in that respect
95 RPL: mmm
96 CAN: the other thing is that without your partner knowing I mean this is in
97      most cases a permanent (.) operation
98 RPL: mmm
99 CAN: which again I said we'll go into in just a minute
100     so it's maybe some things to think about there and we'll go through
        that together
```

At line 91, she points back to what the role-player has just been saying and sums up that this is a '**request**'. But she also conveys her professional *stance* to this request – his request is one that is a little bit outside the norm. She then expands on this with two points that make it unusual. At line 100 she concludes by pointing back to what she has just been saying: 'so it's maybe some things to think about there'. Not only does this summarise the prior talk, but it also describes a way for the listener to interpret this. It gives him a framework for processing what's just been said and what he should do with the information. The points she has made are 'maybe some things to think about', while they talk through the implications of his request. She then does another classic signpost, '... and we'll go through that together', indicating what's coming up later. But again this serves the social function of making it a collaborative, joint task. This collaborative note is quite important given that, throughout this short explanation sequence, she has been indicating a stance that is slightly at odds with the role-played patient's position. 'We' (the GP and role-played patient) will be addressing this unusual request together, making it a joint, shared problem – and not, very importantly, an outright argument between their two positions.

Conveying your professional stance as a GP, particularly when it might not quite align with the patient's view of things, can be a tricky thing to manage. Using this little 'metacommunicative' commentary helps this candidate make her own stance known, to the role-player and to the examiner, without making this argumentative or unprofessional.

### Top tips – metacommunication and signposting

Metacommunication helps any listener interpret what you're saying. But it's especially useful in an OSCE-style exam setting because it gives a commentary for that important overhearing third party, the CSA examiner.

Metacommunication serves lots of functions. Crucially it can serve to help the listener orientate to the structure of your talk and where things are going/what's been said already, a type of metacommunication that's often been termed 'signposting'. This helps your listener understand where things are going and in itself shows that you're attentive to the patient's understanding.

It shows the examiner the structure you are working to, why you are doing something and how attentive you are to patient-centredness. This is a feature of many successful candidates' ways of talking in the CSA.

It might seem like an obvious thing to say, but if you signpost an upcoming part of your consultation, you need to follow through on it. Some of the misunderstandings we identified stemmed from the candidate indicating he or she was going to talk about something, but then going off on a different track, never to return to his or her signposted topic.

Signposting can also serve a more social function, indicating how you want your talk to be interpreted and your position in relation to what's being said. This is especially useful in more complex cases, like Mr J above, but it can be used in routine cases too. For example, telling the patient 'but it's nothing for us to worry about at the moment ...' gives an interpretive framework to understand particular symptoms.

## Physical examinations – giving a good commentary

We've seen that 'signposting' is one important means of metacommunication – pointing to where the talk is going, such as 'can I ask you a few personal questions …', or pointing back, such as '… so that's maybe a few things to think about there'. Commentaries like this are a useful technique to use throughout the consultation, but the research shows that giving a commentary is particularly important when describing physical examinations in the CSA.

Of course, in real life too, it's very important to describe to the patient what the physical exam involves and why it's needed. But not all physical examinations will be carried out 'for real' in the CSA of course; sometimes you will simply get the results on a card. So your commentary becomes even more important in terms of indicating to the role-played patient and the examiner that you know exactly how you would carry out the physical examination.

The next GP struggles with this when he introduces the idea of doing a physical examination.

```
CAN:    alright er now e- (1.2) wh- what I'd like to do
        if that's ok with you I mean er I'll er I'll
        check your pulse your blood pressure right and
        your weight and height if that's ok
RPL:    yes that's fine
CAN:    er and er I mean er a quick er b- abdominal        Candidate requests
        examination just to make sure that I mean you're  physical examination
        not missing any any anything serious there
RPL:    what are you looking for                           Patient question
CAN:    er usually er I mean w- we we we look for any      Candidate's
        any abnormal growth let's say I mean I might       addtional
        like to                                            clarification
RPL:    that sounds quite worrying
CAN:    no it's not at all no er b- I mean I I haven't
        phrased it right I would say er it's just to
        make sure …
```

The candidate starts off quite well, signposting that he would like to move on from data-gathering questions to a few physical examinations:

```
'wh- what I'd like to do if that's ok with you I mean er I'll'
```

and listing some things he'd like to check. However, things get a bit difficult when he asks for:

```
'and er I mean er a quick er b- abdominal examination'
```

without much clarification. The role-played patient asks for a few more details about the examination ('what are you looking for'). This clarification question from the role-played patient is not unusual when talking through a physical examination in the CSA. In fact, we'll see the role-player ask this in the next physical examinations we'll look at. However, your response is quite important. This candidate provides the information:

```
'er usually er I mean w- we we we look for any any abnormal growth let's say
I mean I might like to …'
```

There is some commentary and metacommunication going on here – 'we look for any abnormal growth let's say', but it's not enough and is not quite right. Rather than providing specific information about the examination he will conduct, the 'abnormal growth' is a fairly non-specific piece of extra information about what the examination involves. Worse still, it is likely to cause some anxiety for the role-played patient. So the candidate tries to repair this, metacommunicating that his description wasn't quite right:

`'no it's not at all no er b- I mean I I haven't phrased it right I would say'`

This is metacommunication again, but it doesn't help much here as he's already getting into too much trouble. The candidate then attempts to give some details of what he will be examining. These troublesome sequences can be tricky to repair and in fact this candidate slips up again when describing the physical examination.

So now, let's look at someone who manages the commentary around a physical examination a little better. The candidate we saw earlier in the Mrs T case (see pp. 31–2) had to fit in a forgotten question. After this, he goes on to outline the physical examination he would want to carry out. He outlines this very well, helping him to get the consultation back on track after his earlier, forgotten question.

*Mrs T case – extract 2*

```
CAN:  um (.) sometimes (.) um you can (.) the neck of      Candidate requests
      the womb can kind of come down as well and it it    physical examination
      probably be a good idea for us to have a look to
      make sure that wasn't there (pause) would you be ok
      if I did that with a nurse or would you
RPL:  yeah I mean could you tell me what you're going     Patient question
      to do
CAN:  ok basically want to look at the neck of the womb
      to see whether it's it's coming down as well
      especially I'll I'll be getting you to cough so if
      you cough and the neck of the womb comes down um
      there's other treatments that we could offer like
      a pess- round pessary
RPL:  ok
CAN:  ok it would be a speculum examination               Candidate's
                                                           additional
                                                           clarification
RPL:  that's fine
CAN:  ok so I'll get you to lie up on the couch and I'll
      get the practice nurse to come in with me
RPL:  sure
CAN:  ok
E:    you assume chaperone is present dipstick urine is
      negative
CAN:  thank you very much (.) alright (.)
```

You can see that he gives a much more specific, full account of what the physical examination would involve than the first candidate did:

```
CAN:  ok basically want to look at the neck of the womb to see whether
      it's it's coming down as well especially I'll I'll be getting
      you to cough so if you cough and the neck of the womb comes down
      um there's other treatments that we could offer like  a pess- round
      pessary
RPL:  ok
CAN:  ok it would be a speculum examination
RPL:  that's fine
CAN:  ok so I'll get you to lie up on the couch and I'll get the practice
      nurse to come in with me
```

Giving a full outline of what the physical examination will involve appears to be advantageous to the whole sequence flowing smoothly. Of course, this intimate physical examination cannot be carried out in the exam and instead he is given a card with the results. Giving a commentary is good practice then, but it's especially helpful in an exam setting where you need to demonstrate that you know what you're doing – and what you would be performing if you were carrying out the examination for real.

It can be tricky in a simulation. Even high-performing candidates experienced moments of communicative trouble around physical examinations in the data we collected from the CSA. It can be a tough part to manage entirely smoothly in a simulated, OSCE-style assessment. Don't panic if things go wrong in the physical exam; it doesn't mean the whole consultation is going badly. The ideas about giving a good commentary around your physical exam are worth trying, but it won't spell disaster if there's a bit of confusion.

## Giving explanations

You probably already have a rough idea of what we mean by an 'explanation' in the context of a GP consultation. It's some kind of statement or account from the doctor that makes a particular medical condition, concept or treatment option clear to the patient. They can be done in a range of ways and cover any number of different topics, so again there can never be a 'one-size fits all' approach. A few ideas are presented here that can be usefully employed quite generally when giving explanations.

In the majority of routine CSA cases, after you've done all the data-gathering and, if necessary, a physical examination, it's likely you'll need to give a diagnosis, with an explanation of what it means to the patient. We saw in the section on structuring that this explanation phase usually fell on or just after the 'half time' 5:00 minute marker. Of course, not all cases have to follow this standard data-gathering – explanation – discussion of action structure, but the majority in our study did. Even in more complex cases, where the structure became more flexible, explanations were still usually required from the GP at some point during the 10 minutes.

Ideas on how to structure this explanation phase can be particularly useful. Explanation is a phase that requires a particularly large amount of talk from you, as the GP. Our research on the CSA shows it is a part of the consultation where candidates have to do the most talking, with only short responses from the role-player, which encourage you to continue rather than interrupt. Because you are doing most of the talking, it helps to think carefully about how you structure the things you are saying.

Importantly, though, while you are likely to be doing much more talking during explanation phases, successful candidates are still able to relate the information they are giving back to the role-played patient and create a sense of dialogue even when the role-player isn't saying a great deal. This helps create **alignment** (see p. 26) between the GP and role-played patient because it makes the explanation more than simply an abstract medical description – but something directly relevant to the particular patient and all the things he or she has been talking through in the consultation so far. We'll look at some of these ideas in action to make them clearer.

Some of the explanations here are from fairly complex cases, particularly those describing genetic conditions. Not all cases in your CSA will require this complexity of information, although a few will. However, these more difficult cases display features that are common to many explanation types in the research data. Looking at them closely should help when thinking about explanations in lots of different consultations. This module is not, of course, intended as a substitute for the clinical knowledge required to give explanations – but to give some ideas on structuring and communicating your knowledge effectively.

### Telling it like a story

Given that you have to do a lot of the talking during explanations, it's important to structure the whole sequence in a way that's understandable and signals the start and end of this 'talking-heavy' phase. There are a lot of features in successful medical explanations in our research data that show similar structural features to the way we tell stories in everyday speech. Just like explanations, stories in everyday conversations mean that a speaker takes up a lot of the talking time, with only short 'continuation' words from the other speakers, and structures information in a particular sequence.

Classically, the features of conversational stories run in the order shown on Table 5.4.

*Table 5.4* Features of conversational stories

| | |
|---|---|
| Abstract → | **What the story will be about** |
| Events → | **Sets out the scenario and the sequence of events** |
| Resolution → | **How the events worked out** |
| Coda → | **Rounding off the story and describing the relevance for the listener** |

These are the linguistic terms used to describe spoken narrative structure. Don't worry, you don't have to memorise these exactly, and later in this section we'll think about some of these ideas in more straightforward language, which you can use in your consultation. But for now, let's read a transcript from a candidate who follows this pattern in his explanation and see how it links into this terminology.

This extract comes from a CSA case (Mr H) where the patient has come to the GP with a hospital letter suggesting that he come and discuss the condition that his father died from – haemochromatosis. You can see the letter in Appendix III. The candidate also has a hospital letter in the notes, to read before the case starts. The candidate gives several explanation sequences in this consultation in fact, some related to hereditary risk, some related to options for genetic testing. But this first explanation is about the condition haemochromatosis itself, the symptoms and prognosis. It's a minute-long excerpt that you can also see as a video clip in Session 4 of the RCGP's e-learning modules.[4]

In this excerpt, he gives an explanation about the effects of haemochromatosis. He meets all the requirements of the exam in terms of his clinical knowledge around the condition. But importantly he's also able to communicate that knowledge effectively in a case where he's recognised that the patient wants a lot of information. Particularly take a note of how this candidate begins and ends the explanation sequence.

*Mr H case*

```
CAN:    if we talk a bit about
        you know haemo[chromatosis] that
        […]
CAN:    now haemochromatosis
(pause)
CAN:    if I talk about what it does
        […]
CAN:    um there's er a problem with (.) you know something which (.)
        regulates the transporting of iron
        um and when that's faulty it just
        builds up in your system and it
        takes a very long time
RPL:    mmm
CAN:    um but over years if you have very high ↑- iron levels
        it can cause problems which are the things I was asking
        you so it can actually cause it (.)
        it can make you look very tanned
RPL:    mmm
CAN:    it can affect your sugar levels it
        can affect kind of your ability to get an erection it can affect (.)
        your your you you the way your liver works ↘
        and then [event]ually
RPL:             [yeah]
CAN:    can lead to kind of liver failure
        which I understand is what your
        your father suffered from
```

Notice that this patient offers lots of supportive 'mmms' and 'yeahs' during the explanation, but doesn't interrupt. The role-player doesn't start talking again until the end of this explanation. The role-player's picked up on the candidate's opening gambit and understands the he is about to take up some floor time with an explanation. This doesn't mean that a patient can't ask questions afterwards! But it does mean the role-player is likely to give you a bit of floor time before this happens.

The opening and closing features of stories, what we have called '**abstracts**' and '**codas**', are a particularly useful way to start and end, especially to signal that you are about to take up this floor time. This candidate gives an opening abstract, where he signposts that he will be giving an explanation of haemochromatosis. …

```
CAN:    if we talk a bit about
        you know haemo[chromatosis] that
        [...]
CAN:    now haemochromatosis
(pause)
CAN:    if I talk about what it does
```

> Signpost
> '... if we talk ... if I talk about ...'

This kind of opening signals that you are about to start an explanation. Just like when we signal the start of conversational stories, it means that the listener's likely to give you the space needed to get your information across. Again, it's a kind of **metacommunication**, or 'talk about talk' (see pp. 46–7), and the give-away for this is that he explicitly describes his 'talk' and what it will be about. Metacommunication is a really useful way to perform openings and closings.

He also gives a quick **mini-explanation** of the condition as part of the abstract, in the same way many other candidates do in the examples we'll look at later:

```
CAN:    um there's er a problem with (.) you know something which (.)
        regulates the transporting of iron
        um and when that's faulty it just
        builds up in your system
```

He then sets out the idea that there will be a temporal sequencing to his description:

```
CAN:    and it takes a very long time
RPL:    mmm
CAN:    um but over years if you have very high 1- iron levels
        it can cause problems
```

He points back to the structure his questions took, earlier in the consultation. This is a kind of metacommunication – pointing back at something in the talk to help the listener make sense of what's being said:

```
CAN:    which are the things I was asking you
        so it can actually cause it
(pause)
```

He returns to the symptoms he originally asked about in his data-gathering and now gives them a sequence in time within this explanation. This takes the form of a list, with a repetitive structure 'it can ...' and each new symptom or effect of the illness given as a new piece of information:

```
CAN:    um but over years if you have very high 1- iron levels
        it can cause problems which are the things I was asking
        you so it can actually cause it (.)
        it can make you look very tanned
RPL:    mmm
CAN:    it can affect your sugar levels it
        can affect kind of your ability to get an erection it can affect (.)
        your your you you the way your liver works↘
```

It's difficult to see from the transcript, but if you listen to the clip on the e-learning module then you can also hear the intonation he uses when giving the list – each new piece of information ('tanned', 'sugar levels', 'ability to get an erection') is given with a slight rise in pitch, emphasising the new, non-repeated piece of information.[4] Lists are one useful way of giving a lot of related information in one go – in this case the information is related because it has a temporal order, with an eventual conclusion.

```
CAN:    and then [event]ually
RPL:            [yeah]
CAN:    can lead to kind of liver failure
```

The candidate provides a resolution for the events, or, in this case, symptoms, that he has listed. He has already indicated that symptoms can get progressively worse over time. The resolution comes as a kind of euphemism about the eventual death of the patient. It is a rather medically abstracted description, 'liver failure'. However, he moves on from his more abstract description to a summary that relates it back to the patient.

Signalling the end of the explanation sequence further, with a short coda, helps to relate the relevance of that information back to the patient:

```
CAN:    which I understand is what your
        your father suffered from
```

This way of closing off the explanation provides the patient with a relevant point to start talking more again and to voice his own experiences and concerns.

```
RPL:    yes I mean he they
        kind of went through that gamut with him I mean initially
        it was you know diabetes
CAN:    yeah
RPL:    jaundice [then] cirrhosis
CAN:           [sure] yeah
RPL: and you know he's now yeah
```

The first explanation phase has ended, and now the patient can hold the floor for a while. This is the most he has said for over a minute. At this point, the candidate has not even had to explicitly ask about the patient's concerns – just finishing off the explanation by linking it back to the patient's experiences has been sufficient to prompt a response from him, just as it can when we're telling narratives in conversation.

So as an overview, this candidate's explanation structure took the following, narrative-like form:

| | | |
|---|---|---|
| Abstract | What the story/ explanation will be about<br><br>This candidate does this through signposting, followed by a brief definition | CAN: if we talk a bit about<br>CAN: you know haemo[chromatosis] that<br>[…]<br>CAN: now haemochromatosis<br>PPP: (0.7)<br>CAN: if I talk about what it does<br>[…]<br>CAN: um there's er a problem with (.)<br>CAN: you know something which<br>PPP: (0.6)<br>CAN: regulates the transporting of iron |

| Events/ Symptoms | Sets out the scenario and the sequence of events for the listener | PPP: (0.5)<br>CAN: it can make you look very tanned<br>RPL: mmm<br>CAN: it can affect your sugar levels<br>      it can affect kind of your<br>      ability to get an erection it<br>      can affect<br>PPP: (0.5)<br>CAN: your your you you the way your<br>      liver works↘ |
|---|---|---|
| Resolution | How the events conclude/work out | CAN: and then [event]ually<br>RPL:        [yeah]<br>CAN: can lead to kind of liver failure |
| Coda | Rounding off the story and describing the relevance for the listener | CAN: which I understand is what your<br>CAN: your father [suffered from] |

The story structure described might not always work for you or for all types of explanation, but it's a useful way to think out how you can plan giving your information. If all these terms are too complicated to remember when giving an explanation (they are used by linguists who have a lot of time to slow down the talk and look at these structures after all), then it might be easiest just to keep an idea of where you're starting and ending in mind. These are the kinds of 'openings' and 'closings' that help to signal to the patient (or role-player) when you're about to take up lots of floor time with an explanation and when this phase is completed.

The opening and closing features of stories, what we have called 'abstracts' and 'codas' here, can be particularly useful in signalling these quite 'talk-heavy' phases. In fact, you can often find yourself using this structure in all sorts of places, including more complex cases where the usual data-gathering – explanation – discussion of action sequence does not hold. We already looked at one candidate structuring an information sequence like this in the complex case of Mr J. We analysed her lines 90–100 (see Appendix IV) in detail in the section above on metacommunication. She opened up this short explanation sequence by saying:

CAN:    right it's a slightly unusual request

She then gave some information about the patients she has seen in the past requesting a vasectomy and some of the differences his case presents. She then closed this sequence off by relating that information back to this specific patient:

CAN:    so it's maybe some things to think about there and we'll go through
        that together

Again, in this short explanation sequence, we can see that the role-player stays pretty quiet from the candidate's opening 'right, it's a slightly unusual …' to her signalled ending. So openings and closings are useful in this quite practical way, when you need to hold the floor for a few seconds and get your information across. But we also saw that this was a good example of how metacommunication gives the listener a framework for interpreting what's being said and indicates your own stance as a GP. Giving openings and closings therefore helps gives the role-played patient some pointers on how to interpret the explanation, making this otherwise quite monologic explanation phase more interactive.

This structure can also be useful when getting into the discussion of treatment options or possible actions. In fact the haemochromatosis candidate uses it to describe genetic counselling.

---

### Exercise – Explanations

Have a go at giving the haemochromatosis explanation yourself. You can find the letter that the role-played patient has received at the back of this book (Appendix III), so you could try this out as a full role-play with someone standing in for the patient.

Take one of the practice cases you've already tried from the previous exercises. Select one where you think the explanation sequence was particularly tricky or important for the patient. Give yourself about 1–2 minutes to outline an explanation to the patient in a role-play setting.

You might like to record yourself doing this so that you can play it back. If you haven't got a camera to record yourself, ask the person playing the patient to take note of how you open and close the explanation. If you're becoming familiar with using this type of structure, you can give the explanation more than one try.

---

### Identifiers and mini-explanations

Something that you often have to do when giving explanations is present medical terminology in a way that's understandable. Many successful candidates in the CSA give definitions for medical terms using what we've called a 'mini-explanation' structure. This example comes from the Mr H case, which we've just had a look at:

*Mr H case*

```
CAN:    if we talk a bit about you know haemo[chromatosis] that y-
RPL:    mmm
CAN:    it is (.) what we call a um I mean it's a genetic condition
RPL:    mmm
CAN:    um which means it is (.) inherited
```

So the candidate gives a medical term, 'genetic condition', and uses a 'linking phrase' ('which means …') to elaborate what it means (and, particularly, what it means for this specific patient). This is a really useful technique for demonstrating that you're attentive to the patient's understanding. Perhaps (a little bit cynically) it's also a really good technique for an exam, where you show the examiner that you know the correct medical terms plus how you give them a definition. You can also see in this excerpt that a little bit of 'metacommunication' is used to describe the language being used – 'it's what we call' (see pp. 46–7). Flagging up more difficult words in this way can be really helpful in spoken interaction. Lots of other candidates use the same technique.

*Mr R case – extract 2*

```
CAN:    do you know what this p- (.) what this is called
RPL:    no
CAN:    right well this has got a fancy medical name it's called premature
        ejaculation
(pause)
RPL:    right
CAN:    which means (.) ejaculating before time
RPL:    right
CAN:    so that's what it's called and it is it is fairly it is (.) more common
        than we think actually ...
```

*Mrs A case*

```
CAN:    and you'd like to (0.2) to know more about this
RPL:    mmm
CAN:    right (.) now
(pause)
CAN:    it's it's a funny term cystic fibrosis it's it's a congenital disease
        which means that
(pause)
CAN:    kids are born with it
RPL:    mmm
```

It was often used as the opening part to the story structure for a longer explanation, discussed above – what we called the 'abstract' part of the explanation sequence. You don't have to use these exact phrases in your mini-explanations of course, and sometimes it might not be necessary to provide this level of definition. But it can be useful to see the patterns in the ways others do this. The technique is a useful one to think about, especially in the openings of your explanations, but does not have to be used every time. Using this kind of mini-explanation structure can, in itself, show that you're attentive to the relationship with the patient and his or her understanding. But you can also weave the patient's own terminology into these **mini-explanation** structures, as shown below.

## Relating information back to the patient

Although the explanation phase is quite monologic, many candidates use strategies to maintain 'involvement' with the role-player. Of course making the information understandable is part of that involvement. But there is a very clear strategy many candidates use to maintain a sense of dialogue – by using the voice of the patient in the explanation itself. The candidate in the Mr H case does this very clearly when in one of his **mini-explanations** he says:

*Mr H case*

```
C:      now haemochromatosis
(pause)
C:      if I talk about what it does it as you're right you're completely right
        it is too much iron in your blood
```

Again, this is a kind of metacommunication, pointing back to something the patient has already said: 'you're right, you're completely right…'.

| Term | | Definition |
|---|---|---|
| now haemochromatosis (pause) if I talk about what it does |  | you're right you're completely right it is too much iron in your blood |

Communication skills textbooks often suggest using the patient's own terminology in explanations, particularly in talking through complex information or emotionally difficult issues. This can be a great technique in giving information, but it isn't quite what's happening here. You don't always have precise terms from the patient to hand. More often, successful candidates we looked at in the CSA had particular ways of echoing the role-player's own understanding back in explanations, but weaving this in with medical language. This achieves the same effect – using the patient's own voice in the explanation – but in a slightly more complex way. It builds in some useful medical vocabulary, making it a powerful way of giving new medical knowledge to the patient.

We saw this candidate do other things to link the explanation to the prior knowledge and discussion he has already had. So he draws on the role-player's own language while giving new terms and information. We saw this relational work, linking information back to the patient, with the 'coda' at the end of the narrative structure, with 'which I understand is what your father suffered from'. He also made a 'metacommunicative' commentary, pointing back to something that was said earlier in the consultation:

```
CAN:    but over years if you have very high iron levels it can cause problems
        which are the things I was asking you so it can make you look very
        tanned
```

This links the explanation back to the symptom questions asked of the role-player, helping make the links throughout the consultation.

In explanations, the candidate has to manage the patient's uncertainty and anxiety. Expressing risk, responding to anxieties, showing one's own uncertainty and being persuasive all require conveying information other than in an assertive mode. This is done generally through **modal verbs** in **English** such as 'can', 'should', 'might', etc., which also act as softeners to show respect and emphasise asymmetrical power differences between people.

### Explanatory metaphors

Metaphor can be a useful conceptual tool for conveying difficult ideas. We use metaphor all the time in making sense of things that are abstract or difficult to grasp, by finding equivalence in something more concrete and easier to understand. Medicine makes use of metaphor all the time. In the Mr H explanation we looked at, the candidate uses the metaphor of the body as a kind of machine:

```
CAN:    as you're right you're completely right it is too much iron in your
        blood
RPL:    ok
```

```
CAN:    um there's er a problem with (.) you know something which
(pause)
CAN:    regulates the transporting
(pause)
CAN:    of iron
RPL:    right
CAN:    um and when that's faulty it just builds up in your system
        and it takes a very long time
```

Here the body is a 'system' that should regulate its own iron levels but can be 'faulty'. As with other features that show the relationships between information and ideas, metaphors are also a regular means of **alignment**, making talk more informal or light-hearted as it makes concepts more familiar. It's something to be careful with – metaphors of medicine and the body vary culturally and even person to person. Some have suggested that the metaphor of 'the body as a machine' is too impersonal and disease-centred. It seems to work well in this haemochromatosis case for this patient, but keep attuned to how it's being received. What may be useful in one context might not be so useful in another. The writer Susan Sontag talked a lot about the use of metaphor in the description of illness, particularly ideas of battle and war in discussing cancer and AIDS, such as 'losing the fight against cancer'. Sontag reasoned that metaphors of war confuse the patient and mythicise their illness.[6] The same difficulty might arise with the 'body as a machine' metaphor. Some researchers have suggested the need to listen out for the patient's own metaphors and tailor the talk to suit the patient's own concepts and ways of thinking. It's not always possible to do this, but it can be a great idea to build on the patient's own metaphors if you pick up on them. However you introduce metaphors to your explanations, as long as you keep listening to how the role-played patient is receiving the talk you'll be able to adapt your talk accordingly if there are problems.

### Top tips – explanations

In the CSA, candidates usually do most of the talking in the explanations. This makes it worth giving a bit of thought to how you'll structure your talk. It can be quite daunting to hold so much of the speaking time, especially in an exam setting when there's someone listening to you, but structuring this phase well can help you demonstrate the breadth of medical knowledge you have as well as show that you can relate this to the particular patient.

We looked at several ideas for structuring explanations as a kind of story:

- you can signal the start with a short **abstract**, so that everyone understands and **aligns** with the particular task you are carrying out – an explanation where you will do the majority of the talking
- you can then bring it to a close with a story-like **coda**, describing the relevance of the explanation for the role-played patient. The patient then has a good space to bring up his or her own issues and concerns
- **mini-explanation** structures are a useful way of giving definitions of medical terms and actually form the initial **abstract** for the explanation

- it is useful to use all your prior understanding, which you gleaned from asking questions during the data-gathering phase. Pointing back to things that have already been said – '… which are the things I was asking you …' – is a useful type of **metacommunication**, which helps maintain a sense of dialogue during this talking-heavy phase and achieve alignment
- **metaphors** can be useful tools for explaining abstract concepts with more concrete ideas. But also remember to use them carefully – what works for one patient might not be liked by another.

## Closings and buzzers

Closings in real-life consultations can be quite protracted. Many of the skills you use in real life, such as dealing with multiple complaints and last-minute 'doorknob' questions from the patient, are not going to be needed in the CSA. Another area where the CSA is notably different from 'real-life' talk, then, is the buzzer that will sound exactly 10 minutes after the start of your case. At this point the role-player will get up and leave, with the examiner, without much further talk. Sometimes this can happen when you're in the middle of an explanation about a treatment or action plan:

*Miss L case*

```
CAN:    the the beta blocker that we would use for this can cause some side
        effects of lowering the blood pressure
RPL:    right
CAN:    and so if it was making you feel light headed at [all] then we would
        like you to get back
[BUZZER SOUNDS]
RPL:    uh-huh
```

Again the important thing is not to panic if you were in the middle of saying something! There was no pattern which suggested that candidates who get cut off mid-explanation fared better or worse than other candidates. The communicative indicators of high- or poor-performing candidates were tracked back much further in the consultation structure and generally involved those candidates who had poorly structured data-gathering and had to return to questions late on in the consultation. If you have left yourself at least 3 minutes or so to discuss potential action plans and bring up the most salient points first, the chances are you've covered everything you need to in the 10 minutes.

This was particularly the case in those more complex scenarios, such as the Mr J case we've looked at, in which the patient requests a secret vasectomy, or Mrs C, in which a mother would like to continue surreptitiously administering pills to her schizophrenic son. In these cases, you often don't have to come to a fully agreed upon conclusion – although you will need to have done all that work we talked about above indicating your stance and discussing how things can move forward, in a way that doesn't break down into argument. So again, don't worry if you haven't finalised the course of action by the end of the case. You can get full marks for having done all the other important work.

If you've written a prescription for the role-played patient, you should hand this over to him or her before the end of the scenario. But even this candidate, who doesn't have time to write and hand over the prescription before the buzzer, still passes on full marks because she clearly described, earlier in the discussion of action, what she will be prescribing and agreed this with the role-player:

*Mrs N case*

```
CAN:    ok right ok um shall I give you those prescriptions then or
RPL:    yes thank you
CAN:    would that be ok
        (REACHES FOR PRESCRIPTION PAD)
        There's definitely no other questions
RPL:    no thank you
(pause)
CAN:      (WRITES PRESCRIPTION)
(END BUZZER SOUNDS)
RPL:    ok
        (RISES TO LEAVE) thank you
```

So don't be afraid of the buzzer! You are unlikely to lose marks if you've conducted the rest of the consultation well. A few candidates took the opportunity after the buzzer sounds to do a sneaky 'safety-net' statement and to say goodbye to their role-player.

*Mr H case*

```
CAN:    then you'll find that you're you know you won't
(pause)
CAN:    as you you you'll build up naturally will get rid of it
ACT:    right
(END BUZZER SOUNDS)
ACT:    ok
CAN:    you can come back and see me in a week with any questions
ACT:    thank you very much doctor
CAN:    [thank you very much ok]
ACT:    [thank you very much b- bye]
CAN:    thanks bye
```

Again, it doesn't seem to make much difference to people's marks – but there's no harm in doing this anyway!

Occasionally a few candidates finished just before the 10 minutes. For example, the successful candidate from the Mr O case we saw above finished just after 9 minutes 30 seconds:

*Mr O case*

```
RPL:    and then let me know
CAN:    yes yes I'm and I'm going to do that today
RPL:    ok
CAN:    yeah
RPL:    yeah that's fine
```

```
CAN:    ok
RPL:    all right (0.3) thank you doctor
CAN:    thank you very much
RPL:    cheers bye bye
```

If your consultation has come to a natural close, it's fine to finish off the case a bit early. However, this wasn't a frequent occurrence in the data we had from the exam. Most candidates went to the full 10 minutes on each case. Nevertheless, it is perfectly possible to do well finishing the case off early in this way ... and you're still allowed to go and retrieve your role-player if you're still within the 10 minutes and feel you've forgotten something (it's not ideal, but it is allowed!).

### Top tips – saved by the buzzer!

Finishing on the sound buzzer can feel pretty unnatural – well it is unnatural! – for a consultation. Do not to worry about it too much.

If you've played the earlier parts of your consultation well and stuck to the rough structure outlined above then most candidates do very well, regardless of whether or not they finish mid-sentence or mid-explanation at the buzzer.

Try to hand over prescriptions and any other notes before the end, but again don't panic if you don't manage this – you'll be assessed on the content of the 10-minute talk.

## References

1. Neighbour R. *The Inner Consultation: How to Develop an Effective and Intuitive Consulting Style*. 2nd edn. Abingdon: Radcliffe Publishing, 2005.
2. Roberts C, Atkins S, Hawthorne K. *Performance Features in Clinical Skills Assessment: Linguistic and Cultural Factors in the Membership of the Royal College of General Practitioners Examination*. London: King's College London and Centre for Language Discourse and Communication, 2014, www.kcl.ac.uk/sspp/departments/education/research/ldc/publications/MRCGPling/MRCGPling.aspx [accessed 10 April 2015].
3. Kurtz S, Silverman J, Draper J. *Teaching and Learning Communication Skills in Medicine*. 2nd edn. Oxford: Radcliffe Medical Publishers, 2005.
4. RCGP Online Learning Environment. Clinical Skills Assessment. http://elearning.rcgp.org.uk/csa [accessed 2 June 2015].
5. Lloyd M, Bor R. *Communication Skills for Medicine*. Edinburgh: Churchill Livingstone Elsevier, 2009.
6. Sontag S. *Illness as Metaphor and AIDS and its Metaphors*. New York: Picador, 1990. [*Illness as Metaphor* first published as a single essay, New York: Farrar, Straus & Giroux, 1978].

# Part II

# 6 Introduction to practice cases

*Alexandra Rolfe*

This section of the book gives two whole practice circuits as well as 100 short ideas for additional cases (we have called them 'case suggestions'). The circuits have been reviewed by members of the RCGP Clinical Skills Assessment (CSA) case-writing team and many trialled on trainees. As in the real CSA there is a great variety of conditions and complexities to give examples of the case mix that you might expect to find in the exam.

## How to use the cases

The practice circuits can be used either individually or together to practise a whole exam. As in marathon training it would not be wise to start with a whole circuit; start with one case at a time and try to work up to having tried at least half a full circuit before the exam. This will give you a good idea about timings and how tiring the CSA can be.

As previously mentioned it is best to work in a group of at least three people when you are practising so that someone can act as the doctor, someone the patient and the third as the marker. Mark as per the CSA marking guide for each case and try to be very objective. Stop the consultation at 10 minutes, wherever it has got to, and remember that a patient does not have to be out of the room at the end of the 10 minutes for you to get all the marks, but you must have adequately covered all the important areas.

Before you start make sure that you have an area set up like a consulting room with all the equipment you might need close to hand, including an examination couch and a stop watch. If you can bear it record the consultation to analyse later. If possible turn off all sources of distraction such as mobile phones and ask not to be disturbed. If required make up a card with examination findings before the case so it can be passed to the doctor when appropriate.

If you are running a few cases together before stopping to discuss them, make sure that each is marked at the time it is done and don't forget to take a 2-minute break between the cases and, if doing a whole circuit, after the seventh case have a 10-minute break where you get up, walk around, have a drink and something to eat.

The cases will give you the chance to practise what you have learned earlier in the book about linguistics, structuring and the need to remain open minded and adaptable. As mentioned, keep an eye on the clock so that you leave enough time for the clinical management part of the consultation.

Finally, remember that what is written in the patient notes is not always what they will want to talk about; there is not always one right answer to the case, and some will vary depending on how the doctor responds to the role-player patient.

### How to use the case suggestions

As well as the practice cases there are 100 suggestions for CSA scenarios. These are deliberately brief, and in some cases ambiguous to allow them to be used in different ways and contexts. These can be the starting point for making up your own cases. This is by far the best way to learn how to approach the exam, and what examiners are looking for. It will give you greater insight into how the cases are made up and what is actually feasible in a 10-minute consultation (you will be surprised how much can be done in that time). Have a look at the ideas and then spend a bit of time thinking about how they could be expanded; many can take a number of different paths showing how important it is to be open minded when a consultation starts. For example, consider the possible outcomes for headache, incontinence or cough.

### Developing a circuit of cases

If making up more than one case at a time make sure that you have a good variety of cases with at least three physical examinations per 13 case circuit; these can be anything that is feasible to do in a 10-minute consultation and could include Weber/Rinne's tests, visual acuity and fields, or urinalysis, for example, but is unlikely to include any examination that could be uncomfortable for the role-player, such as fundoscopy or blood pressure measurement. Although there will be no intimate examinations on the role-players themselves, in the past models have been used for candidates to demonstrate their examination technique. If appropriate, offer to examine the candidate, making sure you have offered a chaperone and explained the purpose of the examination. Ensure that the person you are practising on is happy to be examined. There should be at least two ethical dilemmas per circuit and a mix of complexity; for example, one case could be about assisted dying and the next an intermittent claudication, which would require a good examination and discussion of risk factors. Make sure there is a lot of variety in ages, genders, socioeconomic groups and occupations. Don't forget to include some home visits and some telephone consultations. Although there should be diversity in ethnicity, all patients will speak good English as the CSA does not, as yet, have time for interpreted consultations. Even if you speak the same language as the role-player you must conduct the consultation in English at all times.

### Writing cases

Start by deciding on the context of the station – what are you looking for the candidate to demonstrate? Is it an ethical dilemma, social problem, challenging clinical problem or are you looking to assess examination technique? Then, give the patient a name, a gender and an age. Make sure that it is appropriate to the case: for example, a 22-year-old is unlikely to have osteoporosis and men are unlikely to want to discuss hormone replacement therapy. Then start to think about a background for the patient: is he or she thin or overweight, does he or she drink, take drugs or smoke? What is the patient's occupation – does he or she have an occupation? Is the patient from a deprived or an affluent background? What is his or her family situation like? Remember that some cases could be carers, relatives or parents. Every case in the CSA case bank is linked to one of the MRCGP curriculum statements, so it would be good practice to consider how and where the case you are writing links to these.[1] The curriculum statements are all on the RCGP website and Dr Ben Riley's book on the MRCGP curriculum contains information about the statements as well as other guidance to all parts of the MRCGP including the Workplace-Based Assessment (WPBA) and Applied Knowledge Test (AKT).[2]

Next, expand the patient's past medical history, if you think that he or she would have one. Add in medications, including timings and doses, that are relevant to the patient's medical problems. Then think about what the patient is trying to get out of the consultation – is he or she mainly after reassurance or does the patient want further investigations. Why has he or she come to the doctor today?

Write a doctor information sheet based on the following headings: name, age, gender, social and family history, past medical history and medications, including allergies. If appropriate, write the last entry in the notes as the patient may be coming in for follow-up rather than a new consultation.

A role-player information sheet should include name, gender, age and background – which should be kept short and be mainly about the patient's social situation, such as who is at home, employment status, diet, alcohol, etc. Follow this with a good opening statement that should be in lay terms (unless you have an expert patient, such as a doctor). Next decide on further information that can be given if requested by the candidate. This is your chance to give the patient a story. This will give more information about the presenting complaints, including any red flags, and may also contain ideas about what the patient is expecting. Occasionally further written information could be given, such as a hospital letter or printout of information about a specific disease. Write a paragraph with the examination findings if appropriate and finish with a paragraph suggesting to the role-player how he or she should respond to the doctor.

The final section is the marking scheme. It is very useful to make a marking scheme based on the three RCGP domains of Data-Gathering, Clinical Management and Interpersonal Skills. Put down positives – for example, ruling out red flags, a good examination, making the correct diagnosis (although a differential will often do), establishing a good rapport and allowing the patient to contribute and guide the consultation. Negative aspects could be missing important medical history, failing to conduct an examination or ignoring the patient's social context. The candidate will not always need to get all the positives and miss all the negatives to do well. The marks are 3 per section to give a total of 9 per case. Looking at the marking schemes of the practice cases will give an idea of how the marking scheme is structured.

## 100 Brief CSA case suggestions

These are based on the RCGP curriculum, but feel free to overlap cases between statements; for example, a diabetes case could also be about healthy people.

## 3.01 Healthy People: Promoting Health and Preventing Disease

- Cardiovascular risk factor modification.
- Request for weight loss surgery.
- Parent refusing immunisation for her child.
- Teenage mother struggling to look after new baby with little support.
- Patient returning to work after a prolonged break due to illness.

## 3.02 Genetics in Primary Care

- Father has diagnosis of Huntington's disease – what does this mean?
- Son has thrombophilia – what is the risk for the next child?
- A family history of breast cancer – do I need genetic testing? Can I test my children?
- Why is my child being tested for diseases at birth? What are they testing for?

## 3.03 Care of Acutely Ill People

- Shortness of breath after a long-haul flight.
- Fever, tachycardia and positive urinalysis – patient refusing hospital admission.
- Acute confusional state in a nursing home patient.
- Staggered paracetamol overdose over the last week.
- Numb, cold feet in a diabetic who smokes.

## 3.04 Care of Children and Young People

- Mother worried as son has said his uncle gets into bed with him.
- Overweight teenager.
- Musculoskeletal pain in adolescent girl.
- Anxiety and low mood in a teenage boy who is a victim of bullying.
- Chronic abdominal pain – mother concerned that nothing is being done.

## 3.05 Care of Older Adults

- Polypharmacy in an 80-year-old woman.
- Early signs of dementia in an 82-year-old man, brought in by wife.
- Positive initial investigations for myeloma – patient does not wish further investigation.
- Daughter attends to discuss care for her mother who is moving from France and is terminally ill.

## 3.06 Women's Health

- Ongoing abdominal pain.
- 56-year-old with increasing urgency and incontinence.
- 76-year-old woman with spotting.
- 60-year-old with pain on intercourse.
- Recurrent miscarriage.

## 3.07 Men's Health

- Increased nocturia and request for prostate specific antigen (PSA) testing.
- One-sided testicular swelling.
- Request for medication for baldness.
- Domestic abuse against a male partner.

## 3.08 Sexual Health

- 15-year-old requesting a termination of pregnancy.
- Erectile dysfunction in a 25-year-old.
- Persistent bleeding in a 25-year-old with a coil.
- Discussion of contraception.
- Patient thinks that they have HIV because boyfriend was cheating on them.

## 3.09 End-of-Life Care

- Palliative care medication.
- Explaining lack of further treatment for patient's cancer.
- Distress and anxiety in carer of patient who is dying.
- Patient with prostate cancer with sudden-onset leg weakness and incontinence.
- Deterioration at home and patient and family wish to stay at home.

## 3.10 Care of People with Mental Health Problems

- Side effects and monitoring of antipsychotic medication.
- Low mood secondary to difficult life situation.
- Depression post-myocardial infarction.
- Patient who attends frequently looking for admission.
- Parent worried about her daughter self-harming.

## 3.11 Care of People with Intellectual Disability

- New diagnosis of Alzheimer's disease.
- Heavy periods in 17-year-old with severe learning difficulties – brought in by carer.
- Patient with Down's syndrome attending for annual check.
- Behavioural change in patient with severe learning difficulties.
- Parents attend worried that their child has autism.

## 3.12 Cardiovascular Health

- New-onset palpitations.
- New diagnosis of hypertension.
- Increasing shortness of breath.
- Family history of sudden death at a young age.
- Recent myocardial infarction requiring resuscitation, including defibrillation.

## 3.13 Digestive Health

- Recurrent rectal bleeding after passing large stools.
- New-onset reflux in patient of 55.
- New-onset abdominal pain and loose stools with some mucus seen.
- Difficulty with swallowing over the last few months.
- Painless jaundice.

## 3.14 Care of People who Misuse Drugs and Alcohol

- Father concerned that his daughter's mother's partner is taking drugs in the house when she is present.
- Alcoholic who wishes to stop drinking – he comes to you with this problem about once a month.
- Patient who used to take intravenous heroin and is back to discuss their hepatitis B results.
- Mother who takes drugs and wishes to stop, but is afraid that if she seeks help her children will be taken away from her.
- Patient with symptoms of taking excessive amounts of legal highs.

## 3.15 Care of People with ENT, Oral and Facial Problems

- Treatment of chronic rhinosinusitis.
- Persistent pain in jaw.
- Loss of sensation on one side of face.
- Patient who has constant ringing in one ear.
- Young man who presents with loss of hearing.

## 3.16 Care of People with Eye Problems

- Sudden painless complete loss of vision.
- Patient requesting to be registered blind, but does not know what her prescription is.
- Unusual symptoms of flashing lights in one part of vision.
- Pain and discharge from eyes.

## 3.17 Care of People with Metabolic Problems

- Patient whose blood results suggest impaired fasting glucose.
- Over-replaced hypothyroidism in patient who wants to take more thyroxine.
- Symptoms suggestive of Cushing's disease.
- New diagnosis of Type 1 diabetes in a 7-year-old – mother asking for further advice as she thinks it means he is going to die.
- Patient asking for a DEXA scan as they think they are at risk of osteoporosis – use of FRAX (or equivalent) score.

## 3.18 Care of People with Neurological Problems

- Young patient with slight memory loss and recent unsteadiness.
- Carer of child with severe cerebral palsy – not coping and worried she might harm the child.
- 25-year-old suffering from migraine.
- 65-year-old with new-onset headache.
- Recent diagnosis of Parkinson's disease – what does this mean for the patient?

## 3.19 Respiratory Health

- Patient with chronic cough and shortness of breath.
- Worsening of asthma – previously well controlled on just salbutamol but just bought a cat.
- Recent diagnosis of lung cancer and patient wishing to talk through options.
- Well patient who had an X-ray for a cough, which has now resolved, but it showed pleural plaques – what does this mean?

## 3.20 Care of People with Musculoskeletal Problems

- Recurrent pain in knees – struggling to work with it and worried about losing job.
- 2-week history of lumbar back pain.
- Patient with arthritis on methotrexate with symptoms of side effects, but does not want to stop medication as making her feel much better.
- Home visit to elderly patient with rheumatoid arthritis who is really struggling at home, has no help, but does not wish for residential care.
- Recent onset of swelling, pain and stiffness in joints in hands – family history of psoriasis and some scalp psoriasis only revealed if candidate specifically asks.

## 3.21 Care of People with Skin Problems

- 14-year-old with mild acne who wishes referral for Roaccutane (isotretinoin).
- 25-year-old with a widespread rash (possibly allergy, guttate psoriasis, etc.).
- Parents asking for treatment for their son's eczema – she has pictures on her phone.
- Elderly patient with chronic widespread itch – nothing to see on examination.
- 34-year-old patient with worsening of their psoriasis.

## References

1. RCGP curriculum. www.rcgp.org.uk/training-exams/gp-curriculum-overview.aspx [accessed 16 January 2015].
2. Riley B, Haynes J, Field S. *The Condensed Curriculum Guide*. 2nd edn. London: RCGP, 2012.

# 7 Practice cases for the CSA – circuit 1

*Alexandra Rolfe*

## Circuit 1/Case 1: Notes for the candidate

*In this station ...*

You are the GP in a surgery

*Case notes for the patient:*

**Name:**  Patricia Murray
**Age:**    45

*Social and family history:*

Patricia lives with her husband, Scott, and her two sons, David and Luke, age 13 and 11. She works as a claims handler for an insurance company. She is a non-smoker and drinks about three glasses of wine per week.

*Past medical history:*

Recent shoulder pain
Two caesarean sections

*Current medication:*

Co-codamol 30/500mg – 1–2 tablets as required for pain
No known drug allergies

*Last entry in records:*

Four months ago – pain in left shoulder. Diagnosed as soft-tissue injury and treated with co-codamol 30/500.
Recent BP 134/86

## Circuit 1/Case 1: Notes for the role-player

**Name:**   Patricia Murray (female)
**Age:**    45 (the candidate may ask for your date of birth – please prepare one)

### Background:

- You are Patricia, a 45-year-old married woman who lives with her husband, Scott, and two children, David, 13, and Luke, 11.
- You work as a claims handler for an insurance company.
- You don't always eat well, drink a lot of coffee and about three glasses of wine per week. You do not smoke.

### Opening statement:

'I need something to help with my headaches.'

### Information to give if asked by the candidate:

- You have suffered from headaches for many years, but they are worse recently.
- The headaches are now daily.
- If asked about the character of the headaches state: 'They feel like a tight band around the front of the head.' They are worse in the evening.
- Severity of headaches is mild to moderate – about 6/10.
- There is no nausea/vomiting or photophobia. No aura. There is no neck pain.
- There is no increase in pain with bending, coughing or exercise.
- If asked about mood state: 'My mood is OK, I am tired and get angry easily. I am can be teary. I find myself snapping at the children.'
- You have not had a recent eye test.
- Co-codamol and ibuprofen helps with pain, as does sleep.
- You have been taking up to four co-codamols per day and also borrowing your husband's supply when yours ran out, which you knew was not really a good idea. You have not taken more than 4 per day at any point.
- Life is very busy; you spend all your time looking after your family and have little time for yourself.
- Your job is busy and stressful. You deal with insurance claims and the clients are often unhappy with your decision and take their frustration out on you. You also have a lot of pressure from your managers to reach money-saving targets.
- You accept that stress might be contributing to your headaches, but don't know what to do about it.
- You don't think that you are depressed. You have no thoughts of self-harm/suicide, feel that your mood is OK and that you are sleeping normally.
- You just want help with the pain; you are not very concerned that there is an underlying serious illness.
- Your shoulder has improved and you have not required medication for it for a while.
- An examination shows no abnormalities.

continued …

### *How to respond to the doctor:*

- You are receptive to sensible advice.
- You would be keen for ideas of how to decrease your stress levels and are interested in therapy other than the medication, but you are not keen to stop all medication without a suitable alternative suggestion.
- You think that a headache diary would be a good idea.
- You are happy to receive reassurance and accept that there is no sinister cause for the headache.

## Circuit 1/Case 1: CSA case marking sheet

### Case name: Patricia Murray

Case title: Chronic Headache
Context for the case: ability to manage tension headache in primary care

### 1. Assessment domain: Data-Gathering, Technical and Assessment Skills
Recognises tension/medication overuse headache and gathers information about underlying causes

*Positive descriptors:*
- Obtains enough information about headache to exclude a serious problem
- Offers appropriate neurological examination including fundoscopy for papilloedema
- Performs brief neck/shoulder examination to assess muscle tenderness and stiffness
- Elicits information about Patricia's family and occupation that places her problems in context
- Finds out how her headache affects her life

*Negative descriptors:*
- Shows little consideration of different diagnoses for headache
- Fails to rule out red-flag causes of headache
- Fails to offer suitable examination
- Does not explore social or psychological aspects of her presentation
- Does not discuss occupation in context of presentation

### 2. Assessment domain: Clinical Management Skills
Manages headache appropriately

*Positive descriptors:*
- Suggests possible causes for her headache
- Offers reassurance and makes practical solutions to managing headache
- Discusses changes in lifestyle that may help relieve headache such as decrease in caffeine/alcohol, exercise, sleep, etc.
- Broaches the subject of possible analgesia overuse
- Discusses the role of stress in headache
- Suggests a headache diary and trial of no painkillers
- Suggests use of other resources, e.g. eye test

*Negative descriptors:*
- Is unable/unwilling to make potential diagnoses
- Does not discuss the possible effect of life pressures on patient's headache
- Misses chance for opportunistic health promotion
- Suggests medical, including stronger analgesia, interventions where simple practical measures are appropriate.
- Offers investigation for reassurance
- No follow-up arrangements are offered

### 3. Assessment domain: Interpersonal Skills
Uses good communication skills to establish rapport and motivate concordance with plan

*Positive descriptors:*
- Provides understandable explanation of the nature of the headaches
- Shows willingness and ability to discuss possible conflict over cause of headache
- Communicates and explains possible solutions
- Understands the difficulty that headaches getting worse then better might cause

*Negative descriptors:*
- Fails to help Patricia understand cause of headaches
- Does not adapt consultation and suggestions about management to Patricia's social context
- Tells patient what to do rather than making a shared management plan
- Shows little visible interest, lacks warmth in voice/manner

## Circuit 1/Case 2: Notes for the candidate

*In this station …*

You are a GP on a home visit

*Case notes for the patient:*

**Name:**  Evelyn Pritchard
**Age:**     88

*Social and family history:*

Patient is entering the final phase of her illness. She is competent to make decisions. She is being looked after by her daughter, Veronica. She feels that she has had a good life and is not afraid of death.

*Past medical history:*

Patient has been suffering from metastatic breast cancer for five years. Treatment is now palliative.
Osteoporosis – 20 years
Angina – 10 years

*Current medication:*

No known drug allergies
Oramorph 2.5 ml (5 mg) four times daily
Paracetamol 500 mg two tabs four times daily
Alendronic acid 70 mg once weekly
Simvastatin 40 mg nightly
Ramipril 5 mg daily
Aspirin 75 mg daily
GTN spray 2 puffs as required
Adcal D3 two tablets daily

*Last entry in records:*

One week ago. Increase in pain with co-codamol. Still mobile, but becoming frailer and losing weight. Recently seen by a different GP who suggested oramorph for pain.

## Circuit 1/Case 2: Notes for the role-player

**Name:**  Evelyn Pritchard (female)
**Age:**   88 (the candidate may ask for your date of birth – please prepare one)

### Background:

- You were diagnosed with breast cancer five years ago and underwent a mastectomy and had radiotherapy following this. You were given tamoxifen, which you took for three years after.
- Last year you noticed pain in your back and after a trial of painkillers had a scan, which showed cancer in the back as well.
- You live with your husband in a bungalow but you struggle to get about.
- However, you have very good support from your family, especially your daughter Veronica who lives close by and visits almost every day. You feel weak and can find it difficult to keep eating and drinking.

### Opening statement:

'Doctor, my back is really killing me … and I have finished all my tablets.'

### Information to give if asked by the candidate:

- You mainly suffer from pain in the back at the level of the lower ribs.
- The pain is moderate to severe and worse on moving.
- There are no bladder problems, but you suffer from constipation due to the medication, although this has not worsened. You are able to walk. You occasionally feel sick. You do not suffer from headaches.
- You struggle to keep your weight up as you are just not very hungry.
- You have other aches and pains, but there is very little other pain that you worry about.
- You take a lot of tablets that you are unable to remember the names of and are not really sure what they are all for.
- You have had brittle bones for a very long time and have had angina for about ten years.
- Since you were told that there was no more treatment available you have not had contact with any other health professionals except for your own GP, who started you on some form of medication for the pain, but it does not feel strong enough. You have no social care input or private carers.
- You would like more help and advice about what the future will hold and someone to discuss all this with.
- You are a little worried about your husband; he seems to be coping all right, but you do worry that he is hiding his feelings to protect you.

### How to respond to the doctor:

- You would refuse any suggestion of an admission to hospital today.

continued …

- You are very happy to cut down on your tablets and you do not feel that you still need to take tablets for the heart attack or brittle bones. You particularly do not like taking the tablets that you have on a Sunday morning.
- Accept an increase in pain medication even with possible side effects.
- You decline to be examined today as it is uncomfortable.
- Discuss your feelings towards death and that you have accepted it.
- You would welcome the input of the palliative care team and seeing one GP if possible.

## Circuit 1/Case 2: CSA case marking sheet

### Case name: Evelyn Pritchard

Case title: Palliative Care
Context for the case: testing communication skills and awareness of pain management and talking about end-of-life care

### 1. Assessment domain: Data-Gathering, Technical and Assessment Skills
Recognises pain and palliative care as the principal issues and gathers information necessary to understand the patient's situation and offer appropriate help

*Positive descriptors:*
- Obtains enough information to rule out palliative care emergency
- Elicits appropriate information about patient's illness, medical history and medication
- Explores social context of patient and the support she receives from social work, palliative care, etc.
- Gains an insight into the patient's understanding of her illness

*Negative descriptors:*
- Fails to recognise the need for palliative care
- Shows no insight into the complexity of case in context of co-morbidities
- Does not explore the main issues of pain and palliative care support
- Does not take time to investigate the patient's social situation and how her family is being affected

### 2. Assessment domain: Clinical Management Skills
Manages pain, medication and instigation of palliative care simultaneously with appropriate interventions

*Positive descriptors:*
- Offers appropriate suggestions for palliative care analgesia
- Uses common sense to rationalise medication
- Takes into account patient's and family's feelings about her illness when deciding on management plan
- Explains the value of palliative care involvement for both medical and social aspects of care
- Addresses need for support for husband and offers suggestions for this
- Arranges follow-up with practice, ideally with one doctor

*Negative descriptors:*
- Does not address analgesia in palliative care context
- Does not take patient's views into account when discussing medication and/or shows no inclination to rationalise current medication
- Suggests invasive procedures/hospital admission when not required
- Does not consider referral to palliative care
- Follow-up arrangements are not appropriate or absent

### 3. Assessment domain: Interpersonal Skills
Uses good communication skills to establish rapport with patient

*Positive descriptors:*
- Shows willingness and ability to approach a difficult palliative care scenario with sensitivity and caring
- Explains management plan in simple terms that patient can follow
- Offers support and gives confidence that support will be available when needed
- Shows awareness of carer's needs
- Works with patient for optimum management

*Negative descriptors:*
- Fails to respond to patient request for pain relief and to decrease medication
- Is not willing to adapt consultation depending on patient's responses
- Fails to work with patients in improving medication regime
- Creates an uncomfortable atmosphere for patient when discussing her end-of-life care

## Circuit 1/Case 3: Notes for the candidate

### In this station ...

You are the GP in a surgery

### Case notes for the patient:

**Name:**  Deepa Joshi
**Age:**    49

### Social and family history:

Patient lives with husband and one daughter, age 23. Two sons have already left home. She works part-time as a healthcare assistant in a nursing home. She is of Indian origin. She eats a vegetarian diet. She drinks no alcohol and does not smoke.

### Past medical history:

Type 2 diabetes – diagnosed two years ago
Obesity – has been on the obesity register since she joined the practice
Hypertension – diagnosed five years ago

### Current medication:

No known drug allergies
Metformin 500 mg three times daily
Ramipril 5 mg once daily
Atorvastatin 20 mg at night

### Last entry in records:

Three weeks ago – saw the practice nurse for her annual diabetes check. BP 125/84, BMI 31. Bloods taken at the time. UE all normal, LFTs – normal, FBC – normal, cholesterol – 4. HbA1C – 49 (20–42).

## Circuit 1/Case 3: Notes for the role-player

**Name:** Deepa Joshi (female)

**Age:** 49 (the candidate may ask for your date of birth – please prepare one)

### Background:

- You are a 49-year-old woman who lives with her husband and one daughter.
- Two sons have already left home and are married.
- You work part-time as a nursing home assistant.
- You have a nice house in a good area and no financial worries. Although you speak Hindi at home your English is very good.

### Opening statement:

'I think that I am going through the menopause as I keep having hot flushes.'

### Information to give if asked by the candidate:

- You think that you are going through the menopause as you have been having symptoms of hot flushes, which last about five minutes and can strike at any time.
- They are significantly affecting your life. You have difficulty sleeping as you get very hot and then very cold as you have kicked the duvet off. At work your uniform becomes very uncomfortable when you feel hot and the nursing home is not very tolerant of you taking breaks to cool down. This is the thing that bothers you the most and would be keen for the hot flushes to be more tolerable.
- Your periods became closer together and over the last year have begun to get further and further apart and are much lighter than they were. Your last period was three months ago.
- You are generally quite well. Although you are trying to eat healthily, you struggle to lose weight.
- You cook a lot and cook most things from scratch as your husband likes proper food, but it does contain a lot of butter. He is also diabetic.
- You do very little exercise and it has not been something that you have ever been interested in.
- As far as you know there is no family history of breast cancer or strokes.
- You have not had a hysterectomy and you have no unexplained vaginal bleeding.
- You also think that you have become quite grumpy and that intercourse has become more painful, and you are less in the mood for it. This bothers your husband more than it bothers you.
- You would be keen for a blood test to confirm that it is the menopause.
- You have discussed this with you friends and are quite keen on something for the symptoms. You have been trying a herbal medicine called black cohosh and are trying to cook more healthy food, especially soy-based food, to help. You don't really know what is out there.
- You would like to know about the risks of medication and keen to have information to think about at home. You have the internet at home.

continued ...

### How to respond to the doctor:

- You are receptive to sensible advice. You are interested in the options and are keen for further information and to have a think about what to do.
- Although you were keen on a blood test, if it is explained in a sensible manner that you do not require one you are happy not to have a test.
- If the doctor is dismissive of the effect of the hot flushes go quiet and fail to engage with him or her.

# Circuit 1/Case 3: CSA case marking sheet

## Case name: Deepa Joshi

Case title: Menopausal Symptoms
Context for the case: testing communication skills and management of menopausal symptoms

### 1. Assessment domain: Data-Gathering, Technical and Assessment Skills
Recognises menopausal symptoms and their treatment with both conventional and alternative therapy as the main theme of the presentation

*Positive descriptors:*
- Obtains enough information about symptoms to confidently diagnose peri-menopausal symptoms
- Enquires about strategies that the patient has tried, including herbal medicine
- Seeks information about how the symptoms affect the patient and her family, and what she is looking for today
- Seeks information about the patient's lifestyle, including diet and exercise

*Negative descriptors:*
- Does not enquire about the patient's presentation in a logical and systematic fashion
- Fails to explore the social and psychological aspects of the presentation to help understand what her agenda is
- Does not ask about strategies the patient has already tried to manage her symptoms, including complementary therapies

### 2. Assessment domain: Clinical Management Skills
Manages menopausal symptoms and lifestyle simultaneously

*Positive descriptors:*
- Offers appropriate advice and reassurance about the symptoms
- Discusses the use of alternative medication – pros and cons of HRT as well as OTC herbal remedies
- Offers advice about weight loss
- Explores how she could increase her level of exercise in an acceptable way to reduce weight
- Discusses continuing contraceptive needs

*Negative descriptors:*
- Offers further investigation for menopausal symptoms
- Offers inappropriate medical/surgical interventions for treatment of menopausal symptoms
- Fails to discuss the evidence for alternative therapies
- Misses chance for opportunistic health promotion
- No follow-up arrangements are offered

### 3. Assessment domain: Interpersonal Skills
Uses good communication skills to establish rapport and motivate concordance with plan

*Positive descriptors:*
- Shows willingness and ability to discuss menopausal symptoms
- Explores patient's agenda, health beliefs and preferences
- Communicates benefits of healthy lifestyle on symptoms and diabetes
- Acknowledges with patient barriers to change
- Uses simple language and checks understanding
- Acts in a non-judgemental manner and takes cultural factors into account

*Negative descriptors:*
- Fails to respond to request for help with flushing
- Does not explore patient concerns and ideas in a sensitive manner
- Does not work with the patient to form a suitable management plan
- Creates an uncomfortable atmosphere for patient regarding her diabetes, lifestyle and weight
- Fails to make the patient aware of the relative risks of different options

## Circuit 1/Case 4: Notes for the candidate

### In this station ...

You are the GP in a surgery

### Case notes for the patient:

**Name:**   Gordon Smith
**Age:**      65

### Social and family history:

Gordon rarely visits the doctor. He smokes about 20 per day and drinks about 21 units per week.

### Past medical history:

None

### Current medication:

None

### Last entry in records:

Last entry in notes was three years ago with foot pain

## Circuit 1/Case 4: Notes for the role-player

**Name:**  Gordon Smith

**Age:**   65 (the candidate may ask for your date of birth – please prepare one)

### Background:

- You are a 65-year-old man.
- You retired two years ago and used to work on the railways; by the time you retired you ran some of the teams that fixed the track at the weekend. Although you would be out on location, you did not do much of the manual work.
- You are usually well and like to walk your two dogs.
- You live with your wife who has also recently retired and you took up walking to try to keep fit, and as an activity to do together.
- You smoke about 20 cigarettes per day and have done for about 50 years. You know it is bad for you, but you do quite enjoy it.
- You have a beer most nights and at the weekend will have some wine with your wife or drink more if you are out with friends. You think this is about the same as other people you know.

### Opening statement:

'My legs get a little sore when I am out walking, but it improves when I stop for a few minutes.'

### Information to give if asked by the candidate:

- You are usually quite active, but recently have begun to develop pain in your legs when you walk for any length of time. The pain is really quite bad. It is worse when you walk uphill and comes on after a couple of hundred metres. The pain improves when you rest.
- This has gradually been worsening over the last few months.
- You are not really sure what is going on and would like it looked at as you do enjoy hill walking.
- You have some history of heart disease in the family. Your dad had a heart attack when he was in his 70s and your brother who is a little older then you has high blood pressure.
- You never visit the doctor as you have never really been unwell and had about three days off in your whole working life.
- You take no regular medication.

### How to respond to the doctor:

- You think that there is nothing very serious going on and are a little shocked that this may all be related to your smoking. This may be the impetus you need to start thinking about giving up.
- You are not going to make any quick decisions today though.
- BMI 32, BP 165/95, heart – no abnormalities detected (candidate does not need to examine; information can be given on a card). Peripheral pulses should be examined – absent foot and popliteal pulses, blood glucose 5.9.

## Circuit 1/Case 4: CSA case marking sheet

**Case name: Gordon Smith**

Case title: Peripheral Vascular Disease
Context for the case: diagnosis and management of peripheral vascular disease

### 1. Assessment domain: Data-Gathering, Technical and Assessment Skills
Recognises the symptoms of peripheral vascular disease and how they may affect the patient

| *Positive descriptors:* | *Negative descriptors:* |
|---|---|
| • Seeks information about possible peripheral vascular disease and potential risk factors including smoking, diet, alcohol, risk of diabetes, etc. | • Fails to gather information about symptoms and determine severity of possible peripheral vascular disease |
| • Gathers enough information to rule out red flags, such as critical limb ischaemia | • Does not explore possible risk factors |
| • Performs suitable examination of the cardiovascular system and peripheral pulses, including offering to do BP and blood glucose | • Does not offer or does a poor examination |
| • Finds out if leg pain is affecting patient from a social and occupational perspective | • Limited attempt to assess patient's social and occupational context |

### 2. Assessment domain: Clinical Management Skills
Manages peripheral vascular disease appropriately

| *Positive descriptors:* | *Negative descriptors:* |
|---|---|
| • Confidently makes a diagnosis of peripheral vascular disease (intermittent claudication) | • Fails to make a suspected diagnosis of peripheral vascular disease |
| • Discusses further investigations required, such as ankle-brachial pressure index (ABPI), blood tests and ECG | • Does not offer further investigations for peripheral vascular disease including bloods and ABPI |
| • Outlines initial treatment of peripheral vascular disease with a supervised exercise programme and medical modification of cardiovascular risk factors in the form of antiplatelet agents, antihypertensives and a statin. These should be prescribed today | • Does not offer suitable treatment options to patient and take his view into account when prescribing |
| • Educates the patient about the need to change his lifestyle and in particular stopping smoking and modification of diet | • Fails to use the opportunity to discuss lifestyle factors with patient |
| • Organises timely follow-up to review bloods and ABPI | • No suggestion of suitable follow-up or referral to smoking cessation services |

continued ...

### 3. Assessment domain: Interpersonal Skills
Uses good communication skills to establish rapport and motivate concordance with plan

*Positive descriptors:*

- Engages with patient and allows him time to describe his symptoms
- Seeks patient's feelings and concerns towards a diagnosis of peripheral vascular disease
- Uses clear and simple language to help patient to understand the possible diagnosis of peripheral vascular disease and the need for medication and lifestyle modification aiming to stop the intermittent claudication from getting worse

*Negative descriptors:*

- Fails to gauge patient's ideas of what is going on and his level of knowledge about cardiovascular disease
- Fails to allow patient time to think about the diagnosis of peripheral vascular disease and help him to understand what it means for him
- Does not work in partnership with patient to devise a management plan that is acceptable to the patient and contains clear outlines for follow-up

## Circuit 1/Case 5: Notes for the candidate

*In this station …*

You are the GP in a surgery

*Case notes for the patient:*

**Name:**   Mark McLean
**Age:**     23

*Social and family history:*

Patient has only recently joined practice – nil known

*Past medical history:*

Asthma since age 11

*Current medication:*

Salbutamol inhaler on repeats – no recent prescriptions

*Last entry in records:*

None

## Circuit 1/Case 5: Notes for the role-player

**Name:**  Mark McLean (male)
**Age:**   23 (the candidate may ask for your date of birth – please prepare one)

### Background:

- You have just started working as an accountant after finishing university and moved in with your girlfriend about six months ago. Things are going well.
- You are usually well, except you have a touch of asthma that does not really bother you much. You only use your inhaler about twice a year after exercise.
- You can't remember when you last saw a doctor.

### Opening statement:

'I have pain when I pee and a strange fluid is coming out my penis.'

### Information to give if asked by the candidate:

- You have recently been on holiday with your friends from university in Turkey. This was a planned 'boys' holiday' for finishing university and starting work. Since arriving back about ten days ago you have noticed increasing pain while you pass urine and there is a strange thick, yellowish discharge. You have not seen any blood.
- You think that you might have an STI because you had unprotected intercourse with one girl in Turkey while you were on holiday.
- You were very drunk and you do not really remember what happened.
- You did not use condoms and have no idea who the girl was.
- You have only had sex with your girlfriend twice since you got back because you began to feel a little worried after the pain started.
- Your girlfriend has not mentioned any problems with discharge or pain.
- If you do have an STI you would like it to be treated without having to tell your girlfriend. You feel quite stupid and guilty for what you have done.
- The relationship that you are in now is going very well and you are keen not to ruin it. Is it possible to get her tested without telling her why?
- If requested – urinalysis is negative and an examination is normal.

### How to respond to the doctor:

- Respond well to medication to treat your symptoms.
- You are quite happy to provide a sample to test for gonorrhoea and chlamydia.
- Appear surprised if the doctor mentions other infections such as HIV or syphilis.
- If the doctor suggests that you tell your girlfriend appear very reluctant as you do not want to ruin the relationship.
- If discussed in an empathetic fashion respond to a plan to think about telling her, but make no firm decision.
- If the doctor appears patronising or judgemental, become defensive and aggressive – you just made one mistake.
- If the doctor does not mention infection to others say, 'I am a bit worried I could pass this on to my girlfriend.'

## Circuit 1/Case 5: CSA case marking sheet

### Case name: Mark McLean

Case title: Sexually Transmitted Infection
Context for the case: testing communication skills and knowledge of STI management

### 1. Assessment domain: Data-Gathering, Technical and Assessment Skills
Recognises symptoms of STI and the reluctance of patient to tell his girlfriend

| Positive descriptors: | Negative descriptors: |
|---|---|
| • Obtains enough information from history and examination to strongly suspect an STI<br>• Elicits information about Mark's social circumstances including relationship status<br>• Broaches the subject of onward transmission without being prompted<br>• Enquires about asthma and its management | • Fails to recognise common symptoms of sexually transmitted infection and fails to explore possible onward transmission<br>• Does not explore social aspects of the consultation<br>• Fails to offer appropriate examination |

### 2. Assessment domain: Clinical Management Skills
Manages possible diagnosis of STI appropriately and considers risk to contacts

| Positive descriptors: | Negative descriptors: |
|---|---|
| • Offers appropriate testing, treatment if appropriate, and possible referral to GUM clinic<br>• Discusses partner testing<br>• Discusses risk of other STIs<br>• Uses opportunity to discuss drinking habits and health promotion of safer sexual practices<br>• Arranges or discusses asthma review<br>• Offers follow-up to review compliance, test of cure if required and partner notification | • Fails to offer testing for likely STI<br>• No comment on testing for partner<br>• Fails to discuss other possible STIs<br>• Misses chance for opportunistic health promotion<br>• No follow-up arrangements/suggestion of referral to GUM offered, especially if waiting for testing before treatment |

### 3. Assessment domain: Interpersonal Skills
Uses good communication skills to establish rapport and motivate concordance with plan

| Positive descriptors: | Negative descriptors: |
|---|---|
| • Shows willingness and ability to discuss an embarrassing/delicate presentation<br>• Develops an agreed management plan with the patient<br>• Communicates reasons for partner testing and future testing<br>• Recognises the potential ethical dilemma of a positive test and not testing girlfriend | • Fails to respond to Mark's worries about passing the infection on to his girlfriend<br>• Is very rigid in consultation style and does not respond to patient's contributions<br>• Instructs the patient rather than discussing options<br>• Creates an uncomfortable atmosphere for Mark and his situation |

## Circuit 1/Case 6: Notes for the candidate

### *In this station ...*

You are the GP in a surgery

### *Case notes for the patient:*

**Name:**  Linda Potter
**Age:**    54

### *Social and family history:*

Linda lives with her husband, Eric, 63, who was diagnosed with early-onset Alzheimer's five years ago, which is now severe. Linda works part-time in a shop when Eric goes to a day centre. Otherwise she rarely leaves him as this makes him very distressed. He only recognises Linda and the day centre carers. Linda and Eric struggle to get by financially. Non-smoker, drinks two large glasses of wine per night.

### *Past medical history:*

1984 – inflammatory bowel disease
2006 – hypertension

### *Current medication:*

No known drug allergies
Bendroflumethiazide 2.5 mg daily
Mesalazine (Pentasa) tablets 500 mg three times daily

### *Last entry in records:*

Three weeks ago – feeling tired and run down, looking after husband with Alzheimer's disease. Poor sleep due to worry about money. Moderate drinker. Discussed sleep hygiene and cutting down on alcohol. BP 135/84. Review four weeks.

## Circuit 1/Case 6: Notes for the role-player

**Name:** Linda Potter (female)
**Age:** 53 (the candidate may ask for your date of birth – please prepare one)

### Background:

- You are the main carer for your husband, who has quite severe Alzheimer's disease.
- You also have a part-time job in a shop when he goes to the day centre three times per week. You are on a zero-hours contract so if you are not there you don't get paid.
- You drink two glasses of wine per night to help you relax and you feel you can't sleep without this.
- You do not smoke.

### Opening statement:

'My left eye has been sore for a day or so.'

### Information to give if asked by the candidate:

- You woke up yesterday with a painful and red left eye. You hoped that it would go away and took some paracetamol for it.
- Today, the pain seems to have worsened and you have noticed that your vision has started to go blurry. It is sore when you move your eye. You have no headache. This has never happened before.
- You are finding that light makes you eye worse and it is difficult to look at bright lights.
- You would like some eye drops to help with the pain and you are in a bit of a hurry, because you need to get back to your husband.
- You had your eyes last checked a couple of months ago and they were fine.
- Although you have suffered from inflammatory bowel disease for 30 years, it has not bothered you for a long time. You take your medication and are no longer under the care of gastroenterology.
- You are worried about your eyesight, but more worried about your husband who does not cope well with changes in routine.
- You are in receipt of carers' allowance and your husband has DLA (or equivalent), but you have no other carers and on questioning do find it hard to cope with looking after everything.
- You have no family close by to look after your husband if you should become ill. You have no children and have few close friends as they have slowly drifted away as your husband became more challenging.
- You feel very tired and run down. You struggle to sleep because you worry about your finances and your husband.
- If examined – your left eye is red with corneal injection, visual acuity is decreased and your eye is painful to move. You don't really like the light shining in it. It keeps watering. (It might be worth having a picture of anterior uveitis for the doctor to see.)

*continued …*

### How to respond to the doctor:

- You refuse to be admitted to hospital now as you cannot leave your husband on his own, but with some persuasion will attend an eye clinic later as your eye hurts. You may be able to ask a neighbour to watch him as he is prone to wandering. You need to be able to get to work tomorrow as, if you do not work, you do not get paid and financially things are tight.
- You are keen to have further carers and support, and would consider further social work care for your husband as you are getting very tired. You do not think that you are depressed. You have no thoughts of self-harm and your mood is OK; you are just very tired.
- You are very defensive when asked about your alcohol intake and say, 'You would drink if you had my life, doctor.' You do not agree to cutting down and do not really want to discuss it.
- You are not concerned about your inflammatory bowel disease as it has not been an issue for a long time and nothing has recently changed.

## Circuit 1/Case 6: CSA case marking sheet

### Case name: Linda Potter

Case title: Acute Red Eye
Context for the case: recognising potentially serious causes of acute red eye and understanding complex social backgrounds

### 1. Assessment domain: Data-Gathering, Technical and Assessment Skills
Recognises the acute red eye as the principal symptom, but acknowledges the social situation

*Positive descriptors:*
- Obtains enough information to suspect a serious cause for an acute red eye
- Examines eye and tests visual acuity
- Elicits information about the patient's social background, her role as a carer and her ability to cope
- Takes a functional history of the inflammatory bowel disease and hypertension, and clarifies patient is well at the moment
- Finds out about the patient's drinking habits

*Negative descriptors:*
- Fails to recognise a potentially serious cause of acute red eye
- Fails to examine eyes/poor examination skills, leaving out important aspects, e.g. visual acuity
- Is disordered in gathering information about her role as a carer and the impact this is having on her life and health
- Poor skills in eliciting the patient's financial and social situation

### 2. Assessment domain: Clinical Management Skills
Manages uveitis and carer role simultaneously with appropriate interventions

*Positive descriptors:*
- Offers appropriate diagnosis and explains need for emergency referral
- Outlines possible management including eye drops and steroids, which may affect driving
- Makes practical suggestions for changes in drinking habits if time allows
- Explores ways to improve social situation with the help of carers' support, social work and voluntary sector

*Negative descriptors:*
- Fails to make likely diagnosis and understand severity of eye symptoms
- Fails to offer emergency referral and/or plan that suits patient's social circumstances
- Misses chance to discuss patient's social circumstances including follow-up or referral to other agencies

### 3. Assessment domain: Interpersonal Skills
Uses good communication skills to establish rapport and motivate concordance with plan

*Positive descriptors:*
- Explains diagnosis and management in an understandable way
- Takes patient's social circumstances into account and allows flexibility in referral timescales as a result
- Communicates benefits of decrease in alcohol without judging

*Negative descriptors:*
- Fails to make shared plan with patient
- Does not help patient to understand the potential severity of her symptoms
- Unable to discuss social situation in an empathetic manner
- Causes patient to become defensive and disengaged when discussing alcohol intake

# Circuit 1/Case 7: Notes for the candidate

*In this station ...*

You are the GP in a surgery

*Case notes for the patient:*

**Name:**  Colin Banks
**Age:**    64

*Social and family history:*

Colin lives with his wife and is a taxi driver. He sometimes also works as a labourer during the day. His wife has mental health problems and is a regular visitor to the practice.

*Past medical history:*

2000 – hypertension
2006 – high cholesterol

*Current medication:*

Bendroflumethiazide 2.5 mg daily
Simvastatin 20 mg daily
No known drug allergies

*Last entry in records:*

Three months ago by practice nurse. BP 144/86. BMI 28.

## Circuit 1/Case 7: Notes for the role-player

**Name:** Colin Banks (male)
**Age:** 64 (the candidate may ask for your date of birth – please prepare one)

### Background:

- You are a 64-year-old taxi driver. It is long hours and you work various shifts.
- As money is short you also work occasionally as a labourer, but find this tiring.
- You worry about money, as things can be a little tight at times.
- You do not smoke, but you do like a nice glass of wine or whisky and have one most nights with your meal. You might have more if you are entertaining, which you do about once a month.

### Opening statement:

'I can't sleep and need some tablets to help.'

### Information to give if asked by the candidate:

- Sleep is a big problem. You struggle to get to sleep and then wake up quite early. Your sleep pattern is variable depending on the shift you are on. It is affecting your concentration at work.
- You would like some sleeping tablets to help. You had them a few years ago and it made a big difference.
- You do not snore. You are only a little overweight. You are not excessively tired during the day and are able to drive with no problems. You don't drop off during the day.
- You are not sure why you are having trouble sleeping at the moment as nothing much has changed. You live with your wife and both your children have left home.
- You enjoy driving, but the shifts are long and you often have to drink energy drinks to keep you going, especially if you are on a late shift. Often you then need to have a couple of large whiskies to help you sleep. This could be four or five times a week.
- You don't have any serious worries at the moment, apart from the 'usual' to do with finance, and you sometimes get up at night to go to the toilet, but this is infrequent and has not been getting any worse recently.
- Apart from this your health is quite good. You do not have any concerns about the amount that you drink, but your wife has suggested that you think about cutting down. If pressed you probably know that you drink more than you should.
- Although you are keen to retire you are beginning to wonder what the future will hold for you. What will you do with all the free time as you have worked hard your whole life?
- You do not think your mood is low. Your appetite is fine, you have no mood swings, you do not feel teary and you have no thoughts of self-harm.

continued ...

### How to respond to the doctor:

- Be quite forceful about your desire for sleeping tablets. You do not want to cut down on the energy drinks and alcohol as you feel it helps your sleeping rather than affecting it.
- If the doctor is insensitive you will start to feel got at and defensive, and say that this is all a 'waste of time'. The last doctor you saw about this was very understanding and gave you some tablets for a few weeks, which helped temporarily. This is all you are asking for this time. You are not a junkie!
- You are still keen for tablets to try to get the sleeping pattern back on track. You would prefer temazepam as you had it before, but will try something else if required. Be a little annoyed if you do not get them.

## Circuit 1/Case 7: CSA case marking sheet

### Case name: Colin Banks

Case title: Request for Sleeping Tablets
Context for the case: testing communication skills and ability to deal with a difficult request

### 1. Assessment domain: Data-Gathering, Technical and Assessment Skills
Recognises the underlying medical and social factors that are affecting the patient's sleeping pattern

*Positive descriptors:*
- Takes a good sleep history focusing on medical and social factors
- Seeks information about alcohol
- Assesses readiness for change
- Places the sleeping problems in context
- Explores patient ideas on what will help with his sleep pattern

*Negative descriptors:*
- Fails to uncover underlying factors for sleep problems
- Does not take history in an organised fashion
- Fails to identify occupation and relevance to presentation
- No exploration of patient's ideas of why he is having trouble sleeping
- Fails to explore how the patient's life is affected by the problem

### 2. Assessment domain: Clinical Management Skills
Manages sleeping problems, request for medication and excess alcohol intake simultaneously

*Positive descriptors:*
- Suggests appropriate sleep hygiene advice
- Identifies harmful drinking and offers alcohol brief intervention and how patient could cut down on alcohol
- Discusses pros and cons of hypnotics and dangers of driving when tired
- Sets appropriate follow-up

*Negative descriptors:*
- Fails to discuss sleep in partnership with patient
- Misses chance for opportunistic health promotion regarding alcohol
- Suggests medication too easily without taking risks (such as driving) into account
- No follow-up arrangements are offered

### 3. Assessment domain: Interpersonal Skills
Uses good communication skills to establish rapport and motivate concordance with plan

*Positive descriptors:*
- Listens non-judgementally to patient's ideas on causes for his insomnia
- Communicates benefits of cutting down on alcohol and energy drinks
- Enables patient to understand reasons why hypnotics may not be helpful
- Is able to explain reasons in a calm, polite and reasoned manner for reluctance to give hypnotics

*Negative descriptors:*
- Does not give patient time to explain his sleep problems
- Is doctor-centred when discussing management plan and does not allow input from patient
- Creates an uncomfortable atmosphere for patient regarding his request and his problems with alcohol

## Circuit 1/Case 8: Notes for the candidate

*In this station ...*

You are the GP in a surgery

*Case notes for the patient:*

**Name:**  Peter Brown
**Age:**    33

*Social and family history:*

Works as a sales rep and does a lot of travelling. Does not smoke. Limited alcohol intake.

*Past medical history:*

None

*Current medication:*

None

## Circuit 1/Case 8: Notes for the role-player

**Name:**   Peter Brown
**Age:**   33 (the candidate may ask for your date of birth – please prepare one)

### Background:

- You are usually in good health but you developed a sore throat yesterday.
- You are not overweight; you do not smoke and rarely drink alcohol.
- You live with your wife, Sarah, and two boys, Jack and Luke, aged five and two.

### Opening statement:

'I have a sore throat and I need something for it as I am giving an important presentation tomorrow.'

### Information to give if asked by the candidate:

- You were well until yesterday when you noticed your throat was sore. It has worsened over the course of the day.
- You have taken both ibuprofen and paracetamol, which have helped, but you have a very important presentation to give tomorrow and would like it to be gone by then.
- You have also felt a little warm and have a slight dull headache, which is mainly around the front of the head.
- You are not eating much as your throat is sore, but you are trying to keep drinking.
- You are also coughing a bit, but you are not bringing up any sputum.
- Your two children have had something similar and you had to take a day off earlier in the week to look after them.
- You are usually well and rarely visit the doctor. The last time was when you had tonsillitis, which cleared up with antibiotics, about five years ago. You were on holiday at the time and saw an emergency GP at the weekend.
- You would like some antibiotics to get rid of the infection quickly. You would normally sit it out, but this presentation is very important.
- Examination – temperature 37.3, pulse 80, sats 98%, BP 130/85. ENT examination (should be performed): Neck – no cervical lymphadenopathy. Throat – pharynx red and inflamed. Slight tonsillar enlargement and NO pus on tonsils. Ears (should not be performed) – no abnormalities. Chest (should not be performed) – no abnormalities.

### How to respond to the doctor:

- You know that antibiotics are not used as much as before, but you really think that they will help you today.
- You are not keen to leave without antibiotics, but if the doctor explains the reasons for not taking them well you will accept this.
- You would agree to a delayed prescription.

# Circuit 1/Case 8: CSA case marking sheet

## Case name: Peter Brown

Case title: Upper Respiratory Tract Infection and Request for Antibiotics
Context for the case: young salesman requesting an antibiotic for a probable viral sore throat

### 1. Assessment domain: Data-Gathering, Technical and Assessment Skills
Recognises the diagnosis of an upper respiratory tract infection and uses commonly used criteria to assess cause

*Positive descriptors:*
- Obtains appropriate respiratory and ENT history
- Rules out red flags – stridor, difficulty breathing, dehydration
- Identifies patient's agenda – request for antibiotics
- Discusses the presentation in the context of the patient's work pressures
- Conducts good ENT examination including checking for cervical lymphadenopathy, temperature and examining tonsils

*Negative descriptors:*
- Fails to take sufficient history to make likely diagnosis of a viral infection
- Does not offer examination/poorly conducted examination, which will not allow use of CENTOR criteria for diagnosis of sore throat
- No enquiry into the patient's social circumstances, especially occupation and family

### 2. Assessment domain: Clinical Management Skills
Manages URTI appropriately

*Positive descriptors:*
- Gives firm diagnosis of acute pharyngitis
- Explains likely progression and timescale of illness
- Suggests suitable supportive measures including analgesia, avoiding dehydration, use of simple mouthwashes, etc.
- Avoids prescribing antibiotics*

*Negative descriptors:*
- Fails to make diagnosis of likely viral URTI
- Takes a throat swab
- Does not discuss simple supportive measures
- Treats URTI with antibiotics (delayed antibiotics are acceptable)
- Fails to safely net and highlight possible complications of illness

### 3. Assessment domain: Interpersonal Skills
Uses good communication skills to establish rapport with patient

*Positive descriptors:*
- Allows the patient time to explain the reasons for his attendance
- Explains the rationale behind not prescribing antibiotics in a simple and understandable way
- Appears positive rather than defensive regarding the lack of role for antibiotics
- Remains calm and polite when challenged on management options

*Negative descriptors:*
- Fails to listen and discuss patient's expectations
- Is overly patient-centred and gives in to patient demands
- Fails to show good time management skills

* National Institute for Health and Care Excellence. *Respiratory Tract Infections: antibiotic prescribing* (Clinical Guideline 69). London: NICE, 2008, www.nice.org.uk/guidance/cg69/resources/guidance-respiratory-tract-infections-antibiotic-prescribing-pdf [accessed 26 May 2015].

## Circuit 1/Case 9: Notes for the candidate

*In this station ...*

You are the GP in a surgery

*Case notes for the patient:*

**Name:**  Ryan Smith
**Age:**    22

*Social and family history:*

Single, works as a joiner.

*Past medical history:*

Iritis two years ago

*Current medication:*

None

## Circuit 1/Case 9: Notes for the role-player

**Name:**  Ryan Smith

**Age:**    22 (the candidate may ask for your date of birth – please prepare one)

### Background:

- You are a 22-year-old man who lives at home with his parents.
- You work as a joiner.
- You do not smoke.

### Opening statement:

'I am struggling with my back.'

### Information to give if asked by the candidate:

- You are normally in good health, but over the last three months have noticed that you are waking up in the morning with pain in your lower back.
- Your back, as well as feeling sore, can also be quite stiff, which has been annoying you as it is difficult to put your socks on.
- It improves after about an hour and is significantly better with ibuprofen but still a problem. You take 400 mg twice daily.
- You are unable to think of any specific cause for it.
- You had a problem with your eye a couple of years ago, but can't remember what this was, although you were seen at the eye hospital.
- Some days the ache in your back means you have to take a few breaks and so can get behind in your jobs.
- There are no other medical problems.
- You take no regular medication and are not allergic to anything.
- You are of a healthy weight and enjoy a healthy diet.
- You have no bowel or bladder problems. No numbness in your feet, or between your legs in the perineum.
- You think that your dad may have had some problems with his bowels in the past, but again are not sure what it is. There is no history of joint problems in the family that you know of.
- You would like a prescription today to help with the pain as, although ibuprofen is good, the pain has not completely gone.
- You are happy to be examined – the examination shows a decreased range of movement in the back, especially when leaning forward, but no specific tenderness. There are no neurological features in the legs (the doctor should check your legs, feet and tendon reflexes in your knees and ankles).

### How to respond to the doctor:

- Be surprised if it is diagnosed as anything more serious than a muscular problem. However, you would be keen to have further tests and would be interested to know what possible problems the doctor is looking for if he orders further tests.

continued …

- You question if you are able to continue with sport and, if prompted, are keen to know what this means for the future and what the long-term consequences are. Is this going to affect your job?

## Circuit 1/Case 9: CSA case marking sheet

### Case name: Ryan Smith

Case title: Back Pain
Context for the case: testing knowledge of back pain and its management

### 1. Assessment domain: Data-Gathering, Technical and Assessment Skills
Recognises possible causes of back pain from the history and the psychosocial issues surrounding it

*Positive descriptors:*
- Takes suitable history focusing on musculoskeletal and rheumatology systems
- Obtains enough information about back pain to rule out red flags
- Seeks information about occupation/social situation to put back pain into context
- Examines back and legs appropriately – including checking movement and excluding neurological signs

*Negative descriptors:*
- Fails to take focused history of pain and rule out red flags
- Does not explore how the pain is affecting work and ability to exercise
- Fails to undertake back and leg examination or poor examination technique

### 2. Assessment domain: Clinical Management Skills
Manages symptomatic treatment of back pain and investigation of underlying cause simultaneously

*Positive descriptors:*
- Makes and explains the possible diagnoses of mechanical back pain or ankylosing spondylitis and further investigations required
- Offers appropriate symptomatic advice – with medication, NSAIDS and non-medication approaches such as physiotherapy, and if appropriate writes suitable prescription
- Suggests suitable follow-up for patient to review symptoms, discuss results of investigation, and possible referral to a rheumatologist
- Signposts to suitable further resources (e.g. Arthritis UK, occupational therapy, support groups)

*Negative descriptors:*
- Lacks confidence in suggesting possible diagnoses
- Provides poor advice about symptomatic treatment and does not take patient's profession into account
- Offers opioid medication without offering simple measures such as paracetamol and heat packs
- Does not listen to patient's feeling towards possible diagnoses
- No follow-up arrangements are offered, including consideration of possible further investigations and referral

continued ...

### 3. Assessment domain: Interpersonal Skills

Uses good communication skills to establish rapport and allow patient to discuss his presentation

*Positive descriptors:*

- Shows willingness to make a differential diagnosis and discuss with patient
- Communicates possible further investigations and how these will affect the patient's life
- Willing to answer questions patient has about the likely diagnosis
- Explains possible diagnosis and management in a clear, understandable manner

*Negative descriptors:*

- Does not appear engaged with patient or listening to his responses
- Fails to discuss and describe reasons for examination
- Fails to respond to the patient's concerns about how the diagnosis will affect his life or does not allow him the chance to discuss this
- Does not communicate reasons and importance for follow-up

## Circuit 1/Case 10: Notes for the candidate

### *In this station ...*

You are the GP in a surgery

### *Case notes for the patient:*

**Name:**  Ann Jones
**Age:**    48

### *Social and family history:*

Divorced, children have both left home. Not able to work due to ongoing problems with pain in lower back.

### *Past medical history:*

Appendectomy age 21
Laparotomy for chronic pelvic pain age 31
Chronic back pain for ten years
Migraine since age 15
Chronic fatigue for five years
Upper and lower gastrointestinal endoscopies and abdominal and pelvic ultrasound scans all normal in the last three years

### *Current medication:*

400 mg tramadol daily
Pregabalin 150 mg twice daily
Paracetamol – 1 g four times daily
**Allergies:**
Allergic to codeine – vomiting
Allergic to NSAIDs – GI upset

## Circuit 1/Case 10: Notes for the role-player

**Name:** Ann Jones (female)
**Age:** 48 (the candidate may ask for your date of birth – please prepare one)

### Background:

- You have lived alone since you divorced your husband ten years ago.
- Your children have left home and occasionally visit, but they often get at you for moaning so much.
- You are unable to work due to disabilities and money worries you.
- You smoke and rarely drink alcohol.

### Opening statement:

'I have pain in my stomach; I have had it for years and no one is helping me to do anything about it.'

### Information to give if asked by the candidate:

- You have suffered with abdominal pain for many years; the pain is currently no worse than normal, but you are sick of feeling like this.
- The pain feels more like a discomfort in the lower abdomen that can be mild to severe and sometimes worsens after a heavy meal.
- Your bowels are often sluggish and have been for years. You never vomit although you occasionally feel sick. You see no blood in your stools. You have lost no weight and actually might be putting it on.
- The pain stops you going out and you feel reliant on pills.
- It started ever since you had your appendix removed age 21, which was a very distressing experience.
- You have seen multiple doctors who say there is nothing wrong. They do investigations without saying what they are looking for and then don't tell you what is going to happen next, just give you more pills and tell you to go away. You have had enough of it.
- There must be something wrong that is being missed.
- Your diet is not great, but what is the point in a healthy diet as you always feel unwell anyway. The pain stops you doing any exercise. There is no possibility that you could work due to the pain.
- There is no family history of bowel problems. You recently had a smear, which was normal. Your periods are still regular and can be quite heavy and painful, which just makes you feel worse.

### How to respond to the doctor:

- You would appreciate being examined and the examination is normal. (Note: please hand the doctor a card stating that there are no abnormalities – an examination is not required.)

continued ...

- You appreciate someone taking time to talk to you and find out what your concerns are, mainly that there is something wrong with you that nobody can find. You would like to be free of the pain and would be happy to try anything. You are not that keen for further investigation as it always follows the same pattern. You only periodically take the medication as you don't think that it makes much difference.
- You would be quite keen to attend the pain clinic and with a sensible discussion are happy that someone is taking an interest. You feel that this a start, although you remain quite unhappy about how you have been treated over the years.
- Note: try not to focus too much on your past medical history as you are keen to take things forward.

## Circuit 1/Case 10: CSA case marking sheet

### Case name: Ann Jones

Case title: Chronic Pain
Context for the case: difficult case. Main test is of communication skills and taking time to listen to the patient. This is a scenario that is never likely to be solved in one consultation. Rule out red flags. Take into account the patient's context, including family, occupational and social factors.

### 1. Assessment domain: Data-Gathering, Technical and Assessment Skills
Recognises pain and lack of diagnosis/frustration with the medical profession as main issue in consultation

| *Positive descriptors:* | *Negative descriptors:* |
|---|---|
| • Takes appropriate GI, reproductive and pain history<br>• Rules out red flags<br>• Offers abdominal examination<br>• Elicits cultural and social context<br>• Broaches difficulties with previous assessments/investigations with little or no prompting | • Does not take focused history<br>• Little consideration for potentially serious symptoms<br>• Examination not offered<br>• Fails to discuss the effect that the presentation is having on the patient's life<br>• Fails to elicit patient's reason for attending |

### 2. Assessment domain: Clinical Management Skills
Manages chronic problem, taking into account patient knowledge and expectations

| *Positive descriptors:* | *Negative descriptors:* |
|---|---|
| • Discusses patient's previous referral and investigations<br>• Suggests possible diagnoses – including those that may not be shown by investigation<br>• Advises on ways to optimise the patient's medication<br>• Explores patient's feelings towards an onward referral to a pain clinic or similar<br>• Signposts patient towards suitable resources such as online information/pain charities | • Does not discuss possible diagnoses and ignores previous healthcare encounters<br>• Fails to address reason for attending<br>• Does not make suitable management plan for patient and/or discuss medication<br>• Offers highly unrealistic options to patient |

### 3. Assessment domain: Interpersonal Skills
Uses good communication skills to establish rapport and motivate concordance with plan

| *Positive descriptors:* | *Negative descriptors:* |
|---|---|
| • Shows willingness and ability to approach a patient with a difficult relationship with previous healthcare professionals<br>• Shows ability to acknowledge patient's situation and try to understand it<br>• Communicates possible outcomes and offers realistic expectations<br>• Uses understandable language | • Does not explore the patient's understanding of her illness and her social context<br>• Shows annoyance/lack of empathy during consultation<br>• Fails to demonstrate good time-keeping skills and does not acknowledge that the patient may require further consultations |

## Circuit 1/Case 11: Notes for the candidate

*In this station ...*

You are the GP in a surgery

*Case notes for the patient:*

**Name:**   Clifford Abraham
**Age:**     60

*Social and family history:*

Non-smoker. Occasionally drinks alcohol. Patient is of Caribbean descent.

*Past medical history:*

Hypertension for five years

*Current medication:*

No known drug allergies
Ramipril – 2.5 mg daily

*Last entry in records:*

BMI – 32
Blood pressure – 149/86 two weeks ago

## Circuit 1/Case 11: Notes for the role-player

**Name:** Clifford Abraham (male)
**Age:** 60 (the candidate may ask for your date of birth – please prepare one)

### Background:

- You are usually well.
- You work in a factory.
- You think that your diet is currently good, although you do have a sweet tooth.
- You do not really like to exercise much.
- You live with your wife.
- You do not drink much.

### Opening statement:

'I keep having a funny sensation in my chest that my heart is going very fast. It then goes away.'

### Information to give if asked by the candidate:

- You have been suffering for the last few weeks from the occasional sensation of feeling your heart race. These episodes seem to appear from nowhere and you feel that your heart is going very fast. The heartbeat feels very irregular.
- It can last for about a minute or two and then disappear.
- There is no pain, tightness, breathlessness and you have never felt that you will pass out. Onset is not related to exercise or exertion.
- Apart from hypertension and being a little overweight you are generally well.
- You have good blood pressure with the ramipril, which you take every day. As far as you know you have no problems with your heart.
- There is no family history of sudden death, heart disease or strokes. You have not had any recent falls.
- On questioning you snack a lot and eat rather large portions of food. Once a week you have a take-away.
- You are worried because a friend at work died of a heart attack last month and he was very well, and as far as you know took no medication.
- You would like to be examined and the examination will find a normal pulse and normal cardiovascular examination. Blood pressure today is 150/92. Pulse is 84 and regular. (Note – the doctor should feel the pulse, examine the heart and check ankles. Blood pressure is not required.) Hand over a card with the normal findings.

### How to respond to the doctor:

- You are worried by your funny heartbeat and are keen to have a further investigation in the form of an ECG, which you had about five years ago when you were first diagnosed with your hypertension.
- Explain your fears of dying young, especially as your friend did. Engage with the doctor in sorting out your risk factors.

# Circuit 1/Case 11: CSA case marking sheet

## Case name: Clifford Abraham

Case title: Palpitations and Risk Factors for Cardiovascular Disease
Context for the case: assessment of palpitations and suitable cardiovascular examination.
Knows risks for cardiovascular disease and when to refer on. Takes into account the patient's
context, including family, occupational and social factors.

### 1. Assessment domain: Data-Gathering, Technical and Assessment Skills
Recognises patient's fears and risk factors for cardiovascular disease as main issues in
consultation

*Positive descriptors:*
- Obtains enough information about
  palpitations to make a differential
  diagnosis
- Examines cardiovascular system and
  blood pressure
- Elicits information about risk factors for
  cardiovascular disease
- Seeks information about patient's lifestyle
  to put presentation into context

*Negative descriptors:*
- Is disorganised/unsystematic in gathering
  information about palpitations and risk
  factors for cardiovascular disease
- Does not rule out serious complications
  of palpitations including breathlessness,
  chest pain and syncope
- Fails to examine patient or poor
  examination technique
- Fails to explore patient's concerns
  regarding a friend recently dying

### 2. Assessment domain: Clinical Management Skills
Manages palpitations and risk factors for cardiovascular disease appropriately

*Positive descriptors:*
- Offers appropriate advice about
  palpitations
- Arranges ambulatory monitoring to
  document rhythm when symptomatic
- Shows knowledge of cardiovascular risk
  factors and their modification including
  optimisation of blood pressure
- Discusses patient's concerns about heart
  disease
- Suggests patient attend for their bloods
  (FBC, UE, LFTs, TFTs, cholesterol) with
  practice nurse
- Arranges follow-up with results of
  monitoring and blood tests

*Negative descriptors:*
- Fails to suggest possible causes for
  palpitations
- Fails to offer further investigation into
  palpitations
- Misses chance for discussion of
  cardiovascular risk factors
- Does not use opportunity to discuss
  lifestyle factors such as diet/exercise and
  alcohol intake
- No follow-up arrangements are offered

### 3. Assessment domain: Interpersonal Skills
Uses good communication skills to establish rapport and motivate concordance with plan

*Positive descriptors:*
- Finds out patient's concerns about his
  symptoms and what he is looking for
- Is understanding of his fear of dying
- Communicates benefits of improvement
  in lifestyle on cardiovascular risk
  factors with an attempt at motivational
  interviewing
- Explains possible diagnoses and
  management in clear and understandable
  language

*Negative descriptors:*
- Fails to respond to patient's concerns
  about a heart attack
- Performs cardiovascular examination
  without clear explanations of what is
  being examined and why
- Does not explain clearly the reasons for
  further investigation and the importance
  of follow-up

## Circuit 1/Case 12: Notes for the candidate

*In this station ...*

You are the GP in a surgery

*Case notes for the patient:*

**Name:**  Jane McLeish
**Age:**    31

*Social and family history:*

The patient works in an office.

*Past medical history:*

None

*Current medication:*

None

# Circuit 1/Case 12: Notes for the role-player

**Name:**   Jane McLeish (female)
**Age:**   31 (the candidate may ask for your date of birth – please prepare one)

## Background:

- You are eight weeks pregnant with your first child.
- Normally you are well, with no medical problems.
- You work as a medical secretary.
- You have been taking folic acid for the last couple of years and have been careful about what you eat.
- You are currently drinking no alcohol.

## Opening statement:

'I am feeling dreadful, I am eight weeks pregnant and feel awful. I can't keep anything down and am unable to go to work.'

## Information to give if asked by the candidate:

- You and your husband are very pleased that you are pregnant as you have been trying for about three years to get pregnant and are on the waiting list for IVF.
- You have been feeling sick for the last two weeks, but it is getting worse and worse. Even water is making you sick. You can't get to your job as a medical secretary as you are feeling so awful.
- You have also had sore breasts and are very tired. You have only lost a minimal amount of weight.
- Your last period was eight weeks ago and you have had no bleeding or spotting. You have no abdominal pain. You had one miscarriage four years ago. That started with bleeding.
- You have looked online and have been trying various suggestions such as ginger and eating little bits of things often, but it is not helping. You are so fed up.
- You just want to stop feeling so bad. You are not keen for any medication, but realise that it might be required.
- Urinalysis shows a positive pregnancy test and 1+ of ketones. BP is normal. Pulse is normal.
- You are very anxious as it has taken so long to get pregnant and you think that the vomiting might cause another miscarriage.

## How to respond to the doctor:

- You welcome a discussion of possible options and feel worried if you discuss the dangers of becoming dehydrated. You have had friends who have ended up in hospital on a drip and you don't want that to happen to you.
- If offered you would be keen to see how things go over the next 24 hours and are reassured that this is a very common problem.

*continued …*

- You are either happy to take medication as long as the side effects are discussed or come back the following day to have your urine looked at again. You will be quite unhappy to be told there is nothing that can be done and you are just to get on with it.
- You would like the doctor to promise you that you will not lose the baby.

# Circuit 1/Case 12: CSA case marking sheet

## Case name: Jane McLeish

Case title: Vomiting in Pregnancy
Context for the case: test knowledge of common pregnancy symptoms and understanding patient concerns

### 1. Assessment domain: Data-Gathering, Technical and Assessment Skills

Recognises vomiting in pregnancy and underlying fear of miscarriage in patient as main issues in consultation

| Positive descriptors: | Negative descriptors: |
|---|---|
| • Takes appropriate obstetric history including frequency of vomiting and what foods and fluids are tolerated<br>• Rules out hyperemesis gravidarum/severe dehydration or other possible causes of vomiting<br>• Offers urinalysis and blood pressure monitoring | • Fails to takes adequate obstetric/gynaecological history<br>• Fails to offer to undertake urinalysis or blood pressure and pulse<br>• Does not explore the patient's underlying concerns about vomiting in pregnancy<br>• Fails to identify patient's fear of miscarriage |

### 2. Assessment domain: Clinical Management Skills

Manages vomiting in pregnancy and patient's concerns about miscarriage simultaneously

| Positive descriptors: | Negative descriptors: |
|---|---|
| • Reassurance that vomiting is a normal part of pregnancy*<br>• Offers supportive advice of rest and eating little amounts and often. Could also try acupuncture and ginger<br>• Explains what prescriptions (cyclizine or promethazine) could be given if patient is not better and their side effects, and effects on the baby<br>• Early safety-netting and admit if no response to anti-emetics | • Does not discuss vomiting at length and does not offer suggestions for supportive measures<br>• Pushes medical interventions/referral at this point as simple practical measures are appropriate<br>• Does not address patient's underlying concerns about miscarriage and risk of foetal problems<br>• No follow-up arrangements are offered/no safety-netting |

### 3. Assessment domain: Interpersonal Skills

Uses good communication skills to establish rapport and motivate concordance with plan

| Positive descriptors: | Negative descriptors: |
|---|---|
| • Allows the patient the opportunity to discuss her underlying concerns about her vomiting<br>• Discusses low risk of miscarriage and that vomiting is unlikely to cause a miscarriage if treated appropriately<br>• Communicates clearly the different possible approaches to managing presentation<br>• Works in partnership with patient to form a management plan that she is comfortable with | • Dismissive of concerns about vomiting and patient's worries about a miscarriage<br>• Fails to allow patient the opportunity to guide the consultation and make a decision that she is comfortable with<br>• Does not help patient to understand the potential risks of vomiting in pregnancy and the importance of early review of symptoms, whichever management plan is followed |

* National Institute for Health and Care Excellence. Nausea/vomiting in pregnancy (Clinical Knowledge Summary), http://cks.nice.org.uk/nauseavomiting-in-pregnancy#!topicsummary [accessed 26 May 2015].

## Circuit 1/Case 13: Notes for the candidate

### *In this station ...*

You are the GP in a surgery

### *Case notes for the patient:*

**Name:**   Mohamed Sharif
**Age:**   3 months

### *Social and family history:*

Mohamed was born three months ago with no antenatal or neonatal problems. He lives with his mother and father, who are both Muslims.

### *Past medical history:*

None

### *Current medication:*

None

### *Last entry in records:*

Four weeks ago – six-week check normal

## Circuit 1/Case 13: Notes for the role-player

**Name:**   Mohamed Sharif (male)
**Age:**   3 months (the candidate may ask for son's date of birth – please prepare one)

### Background:

- You are Ahmed and you have brought in your 3-month-old son because you would like him to be referred on for a circumcision.
- You are from Pakistan originally, although you have lived in the UK for ten years and would like it done for religious and cultural reasons as all the boys in the family have been circumcised.
- Your wife was born in London and has lived here all her life. She is not very religious, but is a Muslim.
- You attend the mosque on a regular basis.
- Your son will be brought up as a Muslim.
- You state that you wife is also keen for a circumcision although she is not here today.

### Opening statement:

'I would like you to refer Mohamed to be circumcised please.'

### Information to give if asked by the candidate:

- Mohamed is usually well, was born at term and spent no time in the neonatal unit.
- He had a normal 6–8-week check.
- He is your first child.
- On further questioning you mention that your wife is a little unsure about having him circumcised, only because she thinks that it will be painful for him. She understands the religious reasons for circumcision. There are also members of her family who are not circumcised so she does not really understand what the fuss is about.
- However, in your family, if Mohamed is not circumcised he will be looked upon as dirty.
- The child's mother will attend when he has his circumcision.
- You are keen to be able to tell her more about what the procedure will involve and the benefits of it.

### How to respond to the doctor:

- You are at the doctor for one reason only and you will not be happy if you are not referred on for a circumcision.
- If the doctor is adamant that he or she is unable to refer your child to an NHS service state that you wish to have the referral done privately as it is so important to you. You will understand if the doctor has to find out where he or she can refer and get back to you at a later point.
- You will be placated by a referral, but still be annoyed if you are told that there may be a wait as you feel that this is urgent.

## Circuit 1/Case 13: CSA case marking sheet

Case title: Request for Circumcision
Context for the case: knowledge of ethical considerations when referring for circumcision

### 1. Assessment domain: Data-Gathering, Technical and Assessment Skills
Recognises the ethical considerations surrounding circumcision

| Positive descriptors: | Negative descriptors: |
|---|---|
| • Obtains information about reasons for a circumcision in both a cultural and religious context<br>• Seeks information about the health of the baby<br>• Elicits in-depth information about the feelings of both the mother and father towards the circumcision<br>• Explores what the father might do if a referral for circumcision is not given | • Fails to gather information about the background to the request for a circumcision<br>• Does not ask about the wellbeing of the baby<br>• Fails to clarify the mother's feeling towards a circumcision<br>• Fails to ascertain what the father might do if the child is not referred on for a circumcision |

### 2. Assessment domain: Clinical Management Skills
Manages request for circumcision appropriately

| Positive descriptors: | Negative descriptors: |
|---|---|
| • Discusses the local policy towards circumcision for religious reasons – this differs in different areas. Some areas perform circumcisions and some do not<br>• If the doctor does not wish to refer the patient on non-clinical grounds an alternative doctor is suggested<br>• Is able to describe the procedure and possible risks and benefits<br>• Discusses that both parents will be required to attend the hospital when the patient undergoes the circumcision and that they must be in agreement and both sign the consent form | • Refers patient without a full discussion about the risks/benefits and ethical considerations surrounding a circumcision<br>• Refuses to refer patient on for a circumcision for non-clinical reasons without suggesting an alternative doctor<br>• If referring does not describe potential timescale of seeing the hospital specialist and having the procedure done. This is unlikely to be an urgent referral<br>• Fails to discuss the feelings of the mother and the need for her to be in full agreement about the procedure |

continued …

### 3. Assessment domain: Interpersonal Skills
Uses good communication skills to establish rapport and motivate concordance with plan

*Positive descriptors:*
- Acts in a non-judgemental manner and allows the patient time to explain why he is requesting a circumcision for his son
- Discusses sensitively the ethical issues involved and need for the consent of the mother
- Uses understandable terms to discuss the risks and benefits of male circumcision, and clearly explains the next steps
- Ensures the patient is clear about the potential risks of a surgical procedure outwith the NHS
- Remains calm and polite towards father and diffuses potential conflict

*Negative descriptors:*
- Fails to form a positive relationship with the father
- Does not manage to be understanding to his situation while trying to maintain an ethical position
- Becomes hostile and defensive if patient questions the management plan
- Is unable to engage the patient enough to encourage him to attend with the mother
- Is too patient-centred and refers patient on without clear discussion of ethical issues and risk

# 8 Practice cases for the CSA – circuit 2

*Alexandra Rolfe*

## Circuit 2/Case 1: Notes for the candidate

*In this station ...*

You are the GP in a surgery

*Case notes for the patient:*

**Name:** Claire Miller
**Age:** 47

*Social and family history:*

Claire lives with her husband and two children. Her father recently died of bowel cancer.

*Past medical history:*

Depression – diagnosed four years ago
Hypertension – diagnosed five years ago

*Current medication:*

No known drug allergies
Amlodipine 5 mg daily

*Last entry in records:*

Two weeks ago. Seen with increase in loose stools, weight loss, tremor, difficulty sleeping and palpitations. Bloods taken and asked to come back if symptoms not settling. Pulse 94, BP 130/78. Bloods: FBC – normal, UE – normal, LFTs – normal, TSH <0.01 (normal range 0.2–4.0 miu/L), T4 – 29 pmol/L (10–20 pmol/L)

## Circuit 2/Case 1: Notes for the role-player

**Name:**   Claire Miller (female)

**Age:**   47 (the candidate may ask for your date of birth – please prepare one)

### Background:

- You are a 47-year-old woman who recently just does not feel as well as you used to.
- You saw one of the young doctors a week ago and she took some blood tests.
- You live with your husband, two daughters and granddaughter. You spend a lot of your time looking after your granddaughter who is five. She was born when your eldest daughter was 18 and the father is not around. It is because you help that your daughter is able to go to college.

### Opening statement:

'I am just not feeling right and I wanted to know what my blood tests have shown.'

### Information to give if asked by the candidate:

- You have noticed that you have lost weight although you are not eating any less. You are more tired than usual and are struggling to sleep. You seem to have become more restless and irritable.
- You heartbeat feels rapid and you have begun to suffer with loose stools. You have also noticed that you are shaking a little bit.
- This started about two months ago and is worsening, but you do like the fact that people say that you are looking good for the weight loss.
- You came to see one of the doctors two weeks ago but you did not really feel that she knew what she was doing. You thought you would come and see another doctor for the results.
- You are concerned because your father died of bowel cancer and lost a lot of weight as well as having trouble with his bowels before it was diagnosed.
- You think that his illness should have been picked up long before it was, but that many doctors missed it, so you have a little difficulty believing doctors.
- Examination findings – your pulse is 95 and regular, BP 130/85, slight tremor. ENT – small, diffuse, firm goitre. Your eyes are fine and there is nothing else to find on examination.

### How to respond to the doctor:

- Be pleased if they tell you that it is unlikely to be cancer.
- You have heard of the thyroid because you think that your aunt had some problem with her thyroid, which meant she needed an operation.
- Ask for a detailed explanation of the thyroid gland.
- *Prompt* – if the doctor does not ask about your concerns mention that you are scared that you are dying of cancer.

## Circuit 2/Case 1: CSA case marking sheet

### Case name: Claire Miller

Case title: Overactive Thyroid
Context for the case: testing ability to interpret blood results and communicate management

### 1. Assessment domain: Data-Gathering, Technical and Assessment Skills
Recognises thyroid disease as the principal issue but also uncovers negative attitudes towards the medical profession and worries about cancer

*Positive descriptors:*
- Obtains enough information about symptoms to support diagnosis
- Explores possibility of alternative diagnosis including serious illness
- Explores patient's attitude to the medical profession
- Offers to examine thyroid and for other signs of overactive thyroid

*Negative descriptors:*
- Fails or is disorganised/unsystematic in asking about possible symptoms that could be relevant to thyroid disease
- Does not explore psychological aspects of her presentation
- Fails to ascertain patient's attitude to the medical profession
- Does not offer to examine patient

### 2. Assessment domain: Clinical Management Skills
Manages abnormal thyroid function tests and patient's concerns simultaneously

*Positive descriptors:*
- Appropriately interprets thyroid function tests and explains them to patient
- Advises of likely management plan and possible options to treat Graves' disease, such as medical treatments and radioactive iodine
- Advises referral to specialist, but discusses possible treatments for symptoms before she is seen
- Reassures patient that it is unlikely that there is an underlying cancer
- Offers suitable follow-up

*Negative descriptors:*
- Fails to interpret blood results appropriately
- Does not explain the likely referral process for Graves' disease and possible interim treatments
- Does not explore and reassure patient about her cancer worries
- No follow-up arrangements are offered

### 3. Assessment domain: Interpersonal Skills
Uses good communication skills to establish rapport and motivate concordance with plan

*Positive descriptors:*
- Shows willingness to make a diagnosis and explain it in a clear and understandable way
- Explores and discusses patient's ideas and concerns, especially surrounding the belief she may have cancer
- Works with patient to help her regain confidence in the medical profession

*Negative descriptors:*
- Fails to respond to patient's concerns about her symptoms being related to cancer
- Does not help patient to understand her possible diagnosis and the reasons for further referral and treatment
- Does not let patient contribute to the consultation or work with her to develop a management plan

## Circuit 2/Case 2: Notes for the candidate

THIS IS A TELEPHONE CONSULTATION

### In this station ...

You are a GP answering a telephone consultation

### Case notes for the patient:

**Name:** Kelvin Khan
**Age:** 24

### Social and family history:

Kelvin lives alone in social housing. He is known to have had problems with drugs in the past. His father is in prison for assault and his mother, who is also a patient at the practice, tries very hard to help him, but he tends to reject her help. He has a 2-year-old son who he never sees. He is a smoker and unemployed.

### Past medical history:

Known to take cannabis and legal highs.
He was recently seen in A&E after a reaction to a legal high.
He is seen by psychiatry due to possible ADHD as a teenager and ongoing problems with low mood and anxiety. He often misses his appointments.
He was last seen by psychiatry last week, but you do not yet have a copy of this letter.

### Current medication:

None

### Last entry in records:

Two months ago – asking for extension of MED3 for social anxiety. This has been a longstanding problem.

## Circuit 2/Case 2: Notes for the role-player

THIS IS A TELEPHONE CONSULTATION

**Name:** Kelvin Khan

**Age:** 24 (the candidate may ask for your date of birth – please prepare one)

### Background:

- You are the mother of Kelvin, a 24-year-old unemployed male.
- You have phoned the doctor because you are concerned about him.
- You are currently with Kelvin at his flat.

### Opening statement:

'I need help. I am with my son and I think that he is going to kill himself.'

### Information to give if asked by the candidate:

- This morning you have gone round to see Kelvin, who seems very low and is stating that he wants to die. He is just sitting at the window staring out, asking 'What is the point?'
- You are worried that he might actually do something to hurt himself this time as you have never seen him so low.
- You have no idea what has triggered this and he does not seem to know himself.
- Kelvin has struggled with mental health problems, mainly anxiety and possible ADHD, for many years and first saw a psychiatrist when he was still at school. He has never been admitted to hospital before.
- He has self-harmed previously with cutting, but never attempted suicide.
- He recently saw a psychiatrist because of low mood and anxiety. They started him on an antidepressant about a week ago, but you can't remember what it was called and it was given by the hospital pharmacy. He threw the packet away today as he thinks it is useless.
- He has taken drugs and excessive amounts of alcohol for many years and you are always worried about him and have tried many different things to help him. He recently took some form of legal high.
- His physical health is OK, although he does not eat much.
- He has never had a proper job as he feels unable to work due to his mental health problems.
- He has a few friends who are similar to him and as far as you are aware there is no current girlfriend
- He has a 2-year-old son whose mother does not let Kelvin see him.
- He is not willing to speak with a doctor.
- An uncle killed himself a few years ago and Kelvin's dad is in prison for assault.
- You have never known Kelvin to be violent.

continued ...

### *How to respond to the doctor:*

- You are very concerned and anxious; you respond well to a kind and empathetic manner and do calm down a little.
- You need help and you become more anxious if you feel help is not coming.
- Kelvin will speak to you and states, 'What is the point in carrying on?' He sees nothing worth living for and that things are always against him. This new medication has just made things worse.
- He is not keen to see a doctor and will not come down to the surgery, but if a doctor comes to the house he will see them. He will not go to A&E or the local psychiatric hospital.

## Circuit 2/Case 2: CSA case marking sheet

### Case name: Kelvin Khan

Case title: Suicidal Ideation
Context for the case: testing communication skills with a relative of a patient with suicidal ideation

### 1. Assessment domain: Data-Gathering, Technical and Assessment Skills
Recognises the severity of the suicidal ideation and concern of the relative

*Positive descriptors:*
- Obtains enough information about patient to be concerned about the severity of the suicidal ideation
- Assesses risk factors and protective factors
- Tries hard to speak with the patient instead of the mother, to ascertain his thoughts and understanding
- Elicits information about the patient's past medical history including psychiatric and recent drug and alcohol taking

*Negative descriptors:*
- Fails to gain enough information to understand the severity of the suicidal ideation
- Fails to find out about the patient's past medical history and what has happened recently that might have triggered this episode
- Does not explore the social aspects of the presentation
- Significantly breaches confidentially when discussing patient with his mother

### 2. Assessment domain: Clinical Management Skills
Manages suicidal intent and mother's concerns simultaneously

*Positive descriptors:*
- Manages to make a definite plan to get patient seen in a timely manner, taking into account the possible severity of the presentation. This can either be a home visit by the practice or local community mental health team
- Advises mother about not leaving patient alone for any length of time
- Advises mother to phone the police if she feels that she is in danger or the patient is likely to attempt suicide

*Negative descriptors:*
- Fails to arrange suitable immediate face-to-face assessment for patient
- Does not suggest safety-netting measures, both for mother and patient
- Fails to offer any form of follow-up for both mother and patient once acute event is over

### 3. Assessment domain: Interpersonal Skills
Uses good communication skills to establish rapport and motivate concordance with plan

*Positive descriptors:*
- Actively listens to the mother's concerns about her son and his suicide risk
- Reassures and calms mother down
- Is firm, but pleasant, about the need for immediate assessment
- Ensures that management plan is clearly explained including timescale for an assessment

*Negative descriptors:*
- Fails to respond to mother's appeal for help with her son in an understanding and empathetic manner
- Shows a lack of decisiveness in instigating an appropriate management plan in a serious situation
- Does not engage with mother in discussing management plan, ensuring that she has a good understanding and is aware of what to do if the situation deteriorates

## Circuit 2/Case 3: Notes for the candidate

### *In this station ...*

You are the GP in a surgery

### *Case notes for the patient:*

**Name:**  Andrew Hodge
**Age:**    69

### *Social and family history:*

Andrew lives with his wife; both his sons have left home. He is a smoker of about 20 a day. He does not drink alcohol.

### *Past medical history:*

None

### *Current medication:*

No known drug allergies
No prescribed medications

### *Last entry in records:*

Two years ago with cellulitis

## Circuit 2/Case 3: Notes for the role-player

**Name:** Andrew Hodge (male)
**Age:** 59 (the candidate may ask for your date of birth – please prepare one)

### Background:

- You are a 59-year-old postman.
- You are a smoker, about 20 a day, but you do not drink any alcohol.
- Your diet is not very good and you know that you could do with losing a little bit of weight, but your wife is a great cook. You don't do much exercise as you work in the sorting office rather than delivering the mail.
- You do drive, but it is not essential
- You have not visited the GP for a few years as you are usually well.

### Opening statement:

'Three days ago a funny thing happened. I suddenly had problems seeing out my left eye, but it came back after a few minutes.'

### Information to give if asked by the candidate:

- Three days ago you were out walking the dog when the left side of your vision went dull. It was quite sudden and felt as if there was a dimming, as if it had been put in the shade.
- There has been no pain or double vision. There was no headache with it. There were no other symptoms. This has never happened before.
- It must have lasted for about five minutes and then you felt back to normal.
- You are not really very concerned, but your wife told you that you had to come in to get it checked out.
- You are expecting to be told it is nothing to worry about.
- Your father died of a heart attack when he was 72 and your older brother had a heart attack in his mid-60s.
- *Examination* – visual acuity is normal, fundoscopy (normal) and blood pressure (160/95 mmHg) should not be performed, pulse and heart sounds regular and normal. No carotid bruits. BM is normal.

### How to respond to the doctor:

- If asked specifically, you would agree that it was like a curtain coming down over the eye.
- Act very surprised if/when you are told that it could have been a mini-stroke as you feel fine.
- Be accepting of further investigation as you would like to be more in control of your health and you can see how you have let things slide a little.
- Understand why you are not allowed to drive for a month.

## Circuit 2/Case 3: CSA case marking sheet

### Case name: Andrew Hodge

Case title: Amaurosis Fugax
Context for the case: testing diagnostic and examination skills for TIA

### 1. Assessment domain: Data-Gathering, Technical and Assessment Skills
Recognises the possibility of TIA and assesses the main risk factors

*Positive descriptors:*
- Obtains enough information about loss of vision to give differential diagnosis
- Rules out symptoms that need to be seen same day, i.e. ABCD2 score is low
- Seeks information about his risk factors for TIA/amaurosis fugax
- Offers full neurological and ophthalmic examination including blood pressure
- Elicits information about Andrew's occupation to see if this is affected by the possible diagnosis

*Negative descriptors:*
- Fails to recognise symptoms as a possible TIA
- Lack of examination or poor examination skills
- Does not specifically ask patient about his risk factors for cardiovascular disease
- Does not explore patient's occupation and how this could be affected by the diagnosis

### 2. Assessment domain: Clinical Management Skills
Manages TIA, risk factors and driving simultaneously

*Positive descriptors:*
- Suggests suitable referral to TIA clinic as per local guidelines and explains what might happen
- Offers and explains suitable blood tests including FBC, UE, LFTs, ESR, TFTs, cholesterol and blood glucose
- Offers in-house ECG or referral for one
- Suggests antiplatelet therapy – should be given 300 mg aspirin today and then 75mg daily – there are no contraindications
- Organises follow-up including re-assessment of BP in the next 1–2 weeks regardless of referral
- Explains that although he does not need to inform the DVLA as this is the first possible TIA he is not allowed to drive

*Negative descriptors:*
- Fails to refer patient to local TIA service
- Does not offer blood tests and ECG
- Misses chance for opportunistic health promotion
- Does not offer suitable antiplatelet medication
- No follow-up arrangements are offered
- Does not discuss the effects on driving

continued …

### 3. Assessment domain: Interpersonal Skills
Uses good communication skills to establish rapport and motivate concordance with plan

*Positive descriptors:*
- Forms a good rapport with patient, which allows exploration of lifestyle and risk factors for cardiovascular disease
- Explores patient's concerns about the visual loss
- Explains link between visual loss and stroke risk in simple terms
- Sensitively deals with issue of driving
- Motivates patient to attend follow-up appointment and consider changes to lifestyle factors

*Negative descriptors:*
- Does not explore patient's presentation of visual loss and cardiovascular risk factors in a non-judgemental manner
- Does not allow Andrew time to discuss his feelings and concerns about a possible diagnosis of a TIA, its management and the importance of changes in lifestyle
- Explanation of events and management is overly technical or full of jargon

## Circuit 2/Case 4: Notes for the candidate

*In this station ...*

You are the GP in a surgery

*Case notes for the patient:*

**Name:**   Emily Carter
**Age:**     14 years

*Social and family history:*

Emily lives with her mum and is at school. She does not smoke.

*Past medical history:*

None

*Current medication:*

None

*Last entry in records:*

Two months ago with tonsillitis

## Circuit 2/Case 4: Notes for the role-player

**Name:** Emily Carter (female)
**Age:** 14 (the candidate may ask for your date of birth – please prepare one)

*Background:*

- You are a 14-year-old female.
- You live with your mum and your dog, Barney. You are close to your mum, but have not told her that you are coming in today.
- You are currently in fourth year at high school.
- You do not normally drink much, although some of your friends do.
- You do not smoke.

*Opening statement:*

'I had sex two nights ago and I forgot to use a condom. I think that I might need the morning-after pill.'

*Information to give if asked by the candidate:*

- Two nights ago you had sex for the first time and did not use a condom.
- You are now worried that you might be pregnant and would like the morning-after pill.
- You had had a couple of drinks because you were nervous, but knew what you were doing.
- Your partner is 15 and in the year above you at school. It was his first time as well.
- Although you know that it is illegal all your friends are doing it and you think that you love your boyfriend, who you have been with for three months.
- He did not force you in any way or make you drink anything beforehand; he was also nervous.
- You have thought about contraception and after this would be quite keen to take the contraceptive pill.
- You are not overweight and there is no family history of heart disease, stroke or other reasons that might stop you from taking the morning-after pill.
- Your health is otherwise good and your last period, which are regular, was two weeks ago.
- You do not want your mother to know you are here.
- *Prompt* – say 'We are not going to get in trouble, are we?' if the doctor does not discuss the fact that you are underage and your boyfriend is slightly older.
- BP 110/70.

*How to respond to the doctor:*

- You are initially nervous as the whole thing is a little bit embarrassing.
- You are happy to take the morning-after pill and understand the explanation of how it works.

continued ...

- Be angry if the doctor suggests that your boyfriend took advantage of you, or that he should be reported to the police. You were fully aware of what you were doing and will deny it if the doctor takes it any further.
- Appreciate it if the doctor takes the time to discuss contraception in the future as you are keen to discuss this and would be keen to start something straight away.

## Circuit 2/Case 4: CSA case marking sheet

Case name: Emily Carter

Case title: Underage Sex and Emergency Contraception
Context for the case: understanding the ethical issues surrounding underage sex and Gillick/
Fraser competency

### 1. Assessment domain: Data-Gathering, Technical and Assessment Skills
Recognises the ethical issues surrounding the request for emergency contraception

*Positive descriptors:*
- Obtains enough information to be able to make a decision about need for and type of emergency contraception
- Seeks information to make a decision about Gillick/Fraser competency
- Finds out more about the circumstances, including assessing the age difference/position of authority of the partner to see if there are child protection issues
- Explores psychosocial backgrounds and parental awareness

*Negative descriptors:*
- Fails to explore the circumstances of the unprotected sexual intercourse in so far as checking the age and position of authority of the partner
- Fails to establish that the patient meets the criteria for Gillick competency
- Does not explore if the patient was put under pressure to have sex or under significant influence of alcohol and/or drugs
- No discussion of patient's thoughts about contraception for the future

### 2. Assessment domain: Clinical Management Skills
Manages emergency contraception, ethical considerations and future contraception simultaneously

*Positive descriptors:*
- Offers options for emergency contraception
- Explains how the morning-after pill works and what happens if patient is sick
- Discusses the fact that sex under 16 is illegal and why it is illegal, and what it could mean for her partner
- Suggests suitable contraception for the future and explains when this could start
- Broaches the subject of STIs

*Negative descriptors:*
- Fails to offer emergency contraception and/or does not explain how to take it
- Does not broach the ethical dilemmas surrounding underage sex
- Does not discuss suitable contraception for the future or explain how to use it
- Does not inform patient that the morning-after pill will not protect against further risk of pregnancy
- No suggestion of suitable follow-up

### 3. Assessment domain: Interpersonal Skills
Uses good communication skills to establish rapport and motivate concordance with plan

*Positive descriptors:*
- Actively broaches a sensitive issue and helps guide patient to make correct emergency contraception choice for her
- Explores patient's preferences in terms of protecting confidentiality
- Sensitively deals with issue of underage sex
- Motivates patient to consider contraception and in particular long-acting forms

*Negative descriptors:*
- Fails to demonstrate sensitivity and understanding towards patient request for emergency contraception
- Fails to understand that she is nervous and allow patient time to become more confident
- Plans to inform parents against the wishes of patient
- Does not discuss the need for emergency contraception and future contraception in a clear and understandable way

## Circuit 2/Case 5: Notes for the candidate

*In this station ...*

You are the GP in a surgery

*Case notes for the patient:*

**Name:**   Sanjeeta Akram
**Age:**     56

*Social and family history:*

Sanjeeta lives with her husband who is a vascular surgeon. She moved to the UK 20 years ago when he completed his training. She has three children who have all left home.

*Past medical history:*

Hypertension – diagnosed five years ago

*Current medication:*

Ramipril 2.5 mg

*Last entry in records:*

Blood pressure check 135/72 three weeks ago

## Circuit 2/Case 5: Notes for the role-player

**Name:**   Sanjeeta Akram (female)
**Age:**    56 (the candidate may ask for your date of birth – please prepare one)

### Background:

- You are a 56-year-old female.
- You live with your husband who is a vascular surgeon.
- You are a housewife and spend time looking after your grandchildren who are six and four.
- Your diet is vegetarian.
- You do not get outside much and when you do you tend to wear long-sleeved clothes.

### Opening statement:

'I have been feeling tired and my muscles have been aching. My husband thinks I might be low on iron or vitamin D so he would like me to be tested.'

### Information to give if asked by the candidate:

- Your husband has suggested that you come and ask to be tested for iron and vitamin D levels as you have been feeling very tired recently. He is a vascular surgeon.
- You have felt tired for many months but put it down to looking after your two grandchildren twice a week as they are six and four, and very tiring.
- You are tired most of the time, but have felt like this for a long time.
- You have also noticed that you have aching joints and think that your muscles are weaker than they used to be.
- It is mainly the hips and legs that hurt.
- You are slightly overweight, but you have not recently lost any weight, although you do try to from time to time.
- There is no change in bowel habit or problems with passing urine. There is no increased frequency and you are not feeling more thirsty than usual.
- You sleep well and do not feel that you are low in mood.
- You try to eat well, but you and your husband both have a sweet tooth. You eat lots of yoghurt and dairy produce.
- Your husband has a very busy job as a vascular surgeon and works long hours so he is not around to help at home very much. You don't mind this, but it does mean that you don't get to rest much.
- Otherwise you feel quite well.
- There is nothing to find on examination (it does not need to be performed). Urinalysis if suggested is negative and random blood glucose if tested is 5.4.

### How to respond to the doctor:

- You are keen to have your iron and vitamin D levels checked and are quite persuasive in asking for this, especially as your husband is a doctor and wants you to have it.

continued …

- You will be quite unhappy if you do not have the test unless a very good explanation is given.
- You do not really want to start medication without a test.
- You are keen to know what other blood tests that you might have so you can tell your husband.

## Circuit 2/Case 5: CSA case marking sheet

### Case name: Sanjeeta Akram

Case title: Possible Vitamin D Deficiency/Iron Deficiency and Non-specific Symptoms
Context for the case: assessing non-specific symptoms and demonstrating awareness of
possible causes including vitamin D deficiency and iron deficiency, and their management

### 1. Assessment domain: Data-Gathering, Technical and Assessment Skills
Assessment of non-specific symptoms and recognises the potential for vitamin D deficiency
and/or iron deficiency, and further investigation

*Positive descriptors:*
- Obtains enough information about symptoms to make a differential diagnosis including vitamin D/iron deficiency, diabetes, thyroid disease, polymyalgia, depression and fibromyalgia
- Seeks information about lifestyle factors that could potentially cause symptoms, such as diet, exposure to sunlight, etc.
- Offers examination to look for signs that would indicate specific disease such as fever, pulse, blood pressure, muscle tenderness and changes in skin and hair
- Offers urinalysis and blood glucose testing for diabetes

*Negative descriptors:*
- Fails to gather information that would increase the likelihood of a specific diagnosis such as vitamin D/iron deficiency
- Does not explore lifestyle factors that might be relevant
- Fails to consider other causes of being tired all the time and muscle aches
- Does not consider examining patient to look for signs that might help narrow down the potential diagnoses

### 2. Assessment domain: Clinical Management Skills
Manages non-specific symptoms appropriately

*Positive descriptors:*
- Explains that there are a number of possible diagnoses
- Offers blood tests for further investigation into symptoms (FBC, U&E, TFTs, blood glucose, iron levels, calcium, phosphate, LFTs, vitamin D levels and ESR)
- In view of possible diagnosis of vitamin D and/or iron deficiency educates patient about lifestyle changes such as diet and sunlight exposure (30 mins to face and forearms 2–3 times a week, increased if darker skinned) in the summer. Dietary supplementation is required in the winter
- Organises follow-up to assess symptoms and discuss blood results

*Negative descriptors:*
- Fails to discuss the difficulties in making a diagnosis with non-specific symptoms and the need for further investigations
- Fails to consider iron/vitamin D deficiency as a cause of tiredness as suggested by husband
- Does not offer lifestyle advice for vitamin D deficiency as patient is likely to be deficient from history
- Does not give a suitable timescale for follow-up

continued ...

### 3. Assessment domain: Interpersonal Skills
Uses good communication skills to establish rapport and motivate concordance with plan

*Positive descriptors:*
- Assesses the reasons for the patient's presentation today and what she expects to get out of the consultation
- Does not dismiss husband's suggestions of iron deficiency – it is possible – but does not get distracted by it and ignore other possible causes
- Motivates patient to consider lifestyle changes that may help
- Uses understandable language and checks patient's understanding and ability to explain to husband what you think is going on

*Negative descriptors:*
- Fails to allow the patient time to discuss why she is here
- Is rude/undermining about husband's possible diagnosis of iron/vitamin D deficiency
- Fails to involve patient in consultation and help her understand the rationale behind further investigation, and why a definite diagnosis cannot be made today
- Does not offer to discuss presentation with husband if the patient is keen for it

## Circuit 2/Case 6: Notes for the candidate

### In this station ...

You are the GP in a surgery

### Case notes for the patient:

**Name:** John Bell
**Age:** 63

### Social and family history:

Last visit was three years ago with back pain. Smoker. No drugs/alcohol.

### Past medical history:

None

### Current medication:

None

### Last entry in records

Three years ago – mechanical back pain

## Circuit 2/Case 6: Notes for the role-player

**Name:** John Bell (male)
**Age:** 63 (the candidate may ask for your date of birth – please prepare one)

### Background:

- You work as a joiner.
- You still work five days a week, but are thinking about cutting down as you feel more tired than you did before.
- You live at home with your wife who recently retired and she spends a lot of time looking after your grandchildren.
- You smoke about 20 a day and have had no problems from this and do not feel that inclined to stop.

### Opening statement:

'I have a cough and my wife keeps telling me that I have to get it looked at.'

### Information to give if asked by the candidate:

- You developed a cough about two months ago after a cold. It just will not go away and it is beginning to annoy other people.
- It tends to be there all the time and worse when you are working.
- You are not coughing anything up, but feel that you are more short of breath than you were before.
- You have not lost any weight and there is no pain or blood when you cough.
- It does at times wake you up during the night.
- Your cough has actually been going on for a few months and you have been trying to hide it from your family.
- The cough was not worse over the winter and you don't think that you have a wheeze.
- You think that you might have had exposure to asbestos in the past. You have worked with people who have been affected by asbestosis and are aware of the dangers.
- You are also worried about lung cancer and are aware of the risks associated with smoking.
- Otherwise you are well and have barely had a day off work in the last 40 years.
- Both parents died of heart attacks when they were in their seventies.
- Examination – normal respiratory rate. Sats 96%. No clubbing, no cervical LN, slightly decreased AE throughout lungs, no wheeze, chest looks normal.

### How to respond to the doctor:

- You are hoping that the doctor will tell you that it is nothing, but if the doctor offers a X-ray then ask how likely it will be that you have lung cancer and, if you do, what is the prognosis.
- Act upset if the doctor mentions lung cancer, but, if the doctor does not, keep asking if it is a possibility and what the survival rate is likely to be.
- You are not keen to stop smoking from today although you might consider it in the future. You are well aware of the risks.

## Circuit 2/Case 6: CSA case marking sheet

**Case name: John Bell**

Case title: Worsening Cough
Context for the case: testing ability to recognise and appropriately refer 'red flag' symptoms

### 1. Assessment domain: Data-Gathering, Technical and Assessment Skills
Recognises chronic cough and exposure to asbestos and smoking as risk factors for lung cancer

| *Positive descriptors:* | *Negative descriptors:* |
|---|---|
| • Takes good occupational and smoking history<br>• Clarifies nature and duration of cough<br>• Identifies and interprets risk factors for possible lung malignancy<br>• Examines respiratory system appropriately | • Fails to recognise cough as a 'red flag' symptom<br>• Fails to identify smoking and occupational history as risk factors for lung cancer<br>• Does not examine patient<br>• Omits exploration of the patient's socioeconomic context |

### 2. Assessment domain: Clinical Management Skills
Manages urgent referral and follow-up for red-flag symptoms appropriately

| *Positive descriptors:* | *Negative descriptors:* |
|---|---|
| • Follows NICE suspected-cancer referral guidelines*<br>• Suggests urgent referral for chest X-ray, possibly respiratory clinic and spirometry<br>• Makes practical suggestions for smoking cessation<br>• Offers suitable follow-up due to possible sinister cause for symptoms. Even if not serious it is important to follow up to discuss smoking cessation as high risk for lung cancer in future | • Fails to refer patient for further investigation<br>• Misses chance for opportunistic health promotion in smoking cessation<br>• If prompted, fails to discuss possible serious causes for cough<br>• No urgent follow-up arrangements are offered |

### 3. Assessment domain: Interpersonal Skills
Uses good communication skills to establish rapport and motivate concordance with plan

| *Positive descriptors:* | *Negative descriptors:* |
|---|---|
| • Shows willingness to discuss possible serious illness given risk factors for lung cancer<br>• Elicits information about patient's concerns and how this will affect the patient's family life<br>• Communicates and explains benefits of smoking cessation | • Fails to perform in an organised/consistent manner.<br>• Does not discuss the potentially serious nature of the presentation sensitively with patient<br>• Is not understanding of his lack of desire to stop smoking<br>• Shows disproportionate or inappropriate doctor-centredness.<br>• Fails to demonstrate good time management |

* National Institute for Health and Care Excellence. *Referral Guidelines for Suspected Cancer* (Clinical Guideline 27). London: NICE, 2005, www.nice.org.uk/guidance/cg27/resources/guidance-referral-guidelines-for-suspected-cancer-pdf [accessed 15 May 2015].

## Circuit 2/Case 7: Notes for the candidate

*In this station ...*

You are a GP locum in a surgery

*Case notes for the patient:*

**Name:**  Julie Curtis
**Age:**    35

*Social and family history:*

Julie has been at the practice for many years. She joined at the birth of her first child ten years ago. She rarely comes to the practice, just occasionally when one of her children is ill.

*Past medical history:*

Three caesarean sections
Termination of pregnancy aged 18
Anxiety aged 22

*Current medication:*

None

*Last entry in records:*

None

## Circuit 2/Case 7: Notes for the role-player

**Name:**  Julie Curtis (female)
**Age:**    35 (the candidate may ask for your date of birth – please prepare one)

### Background:

- You are Julie, a 35-year-old single mother of three children, aged ten, eight and five.
- You have two jobs, the first working in admin while the children are at school and two nights a week you work in a pub while your mother looks after the children
- Your ex-husband now lives in Australia with his new wife.

### Opening statement:

'For a few months now I have had really bad noises in my ears.'

### Information to give if asked by the candidate:

- You have had ringing in the ears for about three months. It came on quite gradually and seems to be on both sides. It seems to be there all the time. There is no recent trauma to your head or ears.
- It is getting worse and is now beginning to affect your sleep as it is worse when you are lying in bed.
- The sound is like a buzzing with an occasional whoosh. It does not seem to be the same as your heartbeat.
- You do not think that there is any problem with your hearing.
- You do not suffer from headaches, dizziness or nausea.
- When you were younger you used to spend a lot of time in clubs and spent two summers working in the nightclubs in Ibiza. This is where you met your ex-husband.
- There is no family history of ear problems.
- You are always tired and have no time for yourself. You make sure that the children come first, which is why this is the first time you have managed to come in and discuss your ear problems.
- You are otherwise well and take no regular medication.
- You are now beginning to worry that there is something serious going on.

### How to respond to the doctor:

- You are keen for simple measures to try to control the noise.
- You don't really want to go for further investigations as it is difficult to take time off work.
- On questioning you do struggle a bit looking after the family, especially as you have so little time for yourself and spend a lot of time worrying about money. Your ex-husband and father of all the children does not help at all. You don't really know what to do about that and would welcome extra help.
- If questioned in detail about your life start to cry and say that you think you need some help.
- You are keen to have your ears examined (they are normal).

## Circuit 2/Case 7: CSA case marking sheet

### Case name: Julie Curtis

Case title: Tinnitus
Context for the case: assessment of tinnitus in a young woman

### 1. Assessment domain: Data-Gathering, Technical and Assessment Skills
Recognises the presentation of tinnitus and its management in the patient's socioeconomic context

*Positive descriptors:*
- Obtains enough information about presentation to rule out red flags such as unilateral hearing loss, objective tinnitus or tinnitus secondary to trauma or head injury
- Determines if tinnitus is objective or subjective using a stethoscope
- ENT examination including using an otoscope and tuning forks, and assessment of cranial nerves for underlying neurological disease
- Checks for hearing loss
- Elicits information about the patient's socioeconomic context

*Negative descriptors:*
- Fails to gain enough information to rule out potential serious causes of tinnitus
- Does not determine extent of previous noise exposure
- Little enquiry into the social or psychological aspects of tinnitus and how it is affecting the patient's life
- Fails to perform a satisfactory ENT and cranial nerve examination

### 2. Assessment domain: Clinical Management Skills
Manages tinnitus and social considerations concurrently

*Positive descriptors:*
- Makes a definite diagnosis of tinnitus and makes simple suggestions for management
- Suggests referral for formal hearing assessment and to return for blood tests including FBC, TFTs and blood glucose
- Reassures patient that it is likely to get better over time
- Discusses the patient's social situation and suggests ideas for reducing stress and anxiety such as relaxation techniques and exercise
- Signposts patient to suitable resources for tinnitus

*Negative descriptors:*
- Fails to make a diagnosis or relies too much on further testing before committing to a diagnosis
- Fails to advise the patient that the symptoms are most likely to be benign and will improve
- Fails to refer for further testing including a hearing test and blood tests
- Does not address the social circumstances that the patient is in and does not offer suggestions for improvement
- Does not suggest any safety-netting/follow-up for patient

continued …

### 3. Assessment domain: Interpersonal Skills

Uses good communication skills to establish rapport and motivate concordance with plan

*Positive descriptors:*

- Shows willingness to make a confident diagnosis and makes a plan in conjunction with the patient
- Finds out what the patient is hoping to get out of the consultation
- Takes time to address the more challenging aspects of the presentation and manage them in a sensitive manner
- Uses simple and understandable language so that patient is clear about management and follow-up

*Negative descriptors:*

- Fails to engage with the patient and allow her time to discuss the difficulties of being a single parent
- Does not take patient's concerns about tinnitus into account when formulating a management plan
- Explanation of likely causes of tinnitus is confusing or alarming

## Circuit 2/Case 8: Notes for the candidate

### *In this station …*

You are the GP in a surgery

### *Case notes for the patient:*

**Name:**   Thomas Jenkins
**Age:**     85

### *Social and family history:*

Thomas lives alone after his wife died of breast cancer last year; he was the main carer. He does not smoke.

### *Past medical history:*

Myocardial infarction five years ago
Angina for ten years
Atrial fibrillation since the myocardial infarction
Recurrent back pain for 30 years
Hypertension for 20 years

### *Current medication:*

Warfarin – as per INR
Bendroflumethiazide – 2.5 mg daily
Bisoprolol – 7.5 mg daily
Simvastatin – 20 mg at night
Amlodipine – 10 mg
Lisinopril – 2.5 mg
Co-codamol 30/500 – four times daily for pain
Temazepam – 10 mg at night
GTN – two puffs when required for angina

### *Last entry in records:*

Three weeks ago for a chest infection – viral URTI and supportive treatment advised.

## Circuit 2/Case 8: Notes for the role-player

**Name:** Thomas Jenkins
**Age:** 85 (the candidate may ask for your date of birth – please prepare one)

### Background:

- You are a regular visitor to the GP surgery as you have a number of medical problems.
- You live on your own as your wife died a year ago. You have no social work help.
- Your daughter lives close by and often visits.
- You don't smoke, but you do occasionally have a small whisky in the evening.

### Opening statement:

'I have started to feel dizzy when I stand up and a couple of times I have ended up on the floor.'

### Information to give if asked by the candidate:

- Over the last few weeks you have become increasingly unsteady, especially when you stand up and a couple of times you have fallen in the house. The first time you hit the sofa and the second you ended up on the floor, and had to get the ambulance service to come and pick you up. You were not admitted to hospital at that time.
- You are quite worried about this as you are scared of falling. You know friends who have fallen and broken their hips, and then have never been discharged from hospital.
- You suffer from angina, had a heart attack five years ago and suffer from atrial fibrillation
- You take a number of medications for this, but you cannot remember most of them, although you do know that you take warfarin for the irregular heartbeat.
- You are also a bit worried that because you are on warfarin you might bleed a lot if you fall.
- Since your wife died you don't really eat very well as you can't really be bothered cooking now that you are on your own. You are now nervous to go out.
- You currently have no social care input and are able to walk to the shop at the end of the road. You do not have a community alarm. You do not have a dosette box.
- Your daughter lives close by and will often pop in with food. Often it ends up in the bin as you don't eat it before it goes off.
- You don't think that you are depressed, but are a little bit lonely in your house on your own.
- Your back pain does not bother you much, but you take the painkillers as you always have.
- *Examination* – looks thin and pale. BMI 19, lying BP 115/80 and standing 100/70. Pulse – irregularly irregular between 58 and 72. Sats – 98%. ENT – NAD. Neuro – NAD.
- *Prompt* – say 'I am a little worried about falling while I am on the warfarin, doctor.'

continued ...

### *How to respond to the doctor:*

- If sympathetic listen to what the doctor has to say and agree that you might be lonely, and that you have been looking into sheltered housing.
- Agree that your diet is not good and that you would like to eat better. You have lost weight because you are not eating.
- Become more hostile if the doctor focuses on your mood.
- Agree that rationalising your medication would be good as you don't always remember to take it.

## Circuit 2/Case 8: CSA case marking sheet

### Case name: Thomas Jenkins

Case title: Postural Hypotension
Context for the case: diagnosis and management of postural hypotension

### 1. Assessment domain: Data-Gathering, Technical and Assessment Skills
Recognises the presentation of postural hypotension and how to investigate possible causes

*Positive descriptors:*
- Obtains enough information about symptoms to make differential diagnosis
- Enquires about possible risk factors for hypotension, including co-morbidities, medication and social situation
- Seeks information about possible falls risk
- Offers basic examination of patient including vital signs, ENT and neuro (results to be given)
- Rules out symptoms that need to be seen same day
- Seeks information about patient's current home situation

*Negative descriptors:*
- Fails to recognise symptoms as possible postural hypotension
- Does not investigate risk of falls
- Does not explore patient's social situation, in particular the effect of the death of his wife
- Does not offer examination

### 2. Assessment domain: Clinical Management Skills
Manages possible diagnosis and social issues simultaneously

*Positive descriptors:*
- Makes provisional diagnosis of postural hypotension
- Offers blood tests to investigate further including FBC, UE, LFTs, ESR and blood glucose
- Offers in-house ECG or referral for one
- Rationalises medication including reducing/stopping co-codamol and temazepam. Stops at least one antihypertensive – probably bendroflumethiazide
- Refers to community falls team
- Addresses social issues including social work input, change in housing, community alarm
- Arranges suitable follow-up to discuss blood results and effectiveness of rationalisation of medication

*Negative descriptors:*
- Fails to make provisional diagnosis of postural hypotension
- Does not offer further investigations, such as blood tests
- Does not offer rationalisation of medication
- Fails to address social issues including living alone and risk of falls
- Misses chance to discuss diet and other lifestyle factors
- No follow-up arrangements are offered

continued …

### 3. Assessment domain: Interpersonal Skills
Uses good communication skills to establish rapport and motivate concordance with plan

*Positive descriptors:*

- Forms a good rapport with patient that allows exploration of presentation
- Deals delicately with subjects that might upset patient such as loneliness due to loss of wife and low mood
- Sensitively deals with social issues
- Explains diagnosis of postural hypotension and further investigation in a clear and simple manner

*Negative descriptors:*

- Does not adapt consultation to suit patient
- Does not seem interested and empathetic when discussing social context
- Does not form a management plan with Thomas and instead instructs him on what to do
- Does not motivate Thomas to make positive decisions about the future

## Circuit 2/Case 9: Notes for the candidate

*In this station ...*

You are the GP in a surgery

*Case notes for the patient:*

**Name:**  Cheryl Cameron
**Age:**  29

*Social and family history:*

Patient lives with her husband and works as a manager in a shoe shop. She rarely visits the doctor.

*Past medical history:*

None

*Current medication:*

None

*Other clinical details:*

All immunisations up to date

## Circuit 2/Case 9: Notes for the role-player

**Name:**  Cheryl Cameron
**Age:**  29 (the candidate may ask for your date of birth – please prepare one)

### Background:

- Your sister's son (who is six months old) has just been diagnosed with cystic fibrosis, which was picked up on testing just after birth.
- This has been stressful for the family, but not completely unexpected as your uncle had the disease and died age 33 of pneumonia.

### Opening statement:

'My nephew has recently been diagnosed with something called cystic fibrosis. I would like to have children soon and am worried that they might have it.'

### Information to give if asked by the candidate:

- You are feeling well and take no medication apart from folic acid as you are considering pregnancy.
- Your brother, sister and husband are all well. As far as you know there is no cystic fibrosis in your husband's family.
- Your nephew was born early and spent time in the neonatal unit. He still seems quite small.
- You did not know your uncle well as he died just before you were born, but you have been told he had cystic fibrosis, which caused him to have lots of chest infections and he was always ill.
- You are keen to find out more about cystic fibrosis and what symptoms it causes. What does it mean for your nephew?
- Also, you would like to know what the likelihood your children having the disease is.

### How to respond to the doctor:

- You would be surprised if the doctor had not heard of the disease as you think it is quite common.
- You wonder if you could have genetic testing before you became pregnant and, if a carrier, could the baby be screened before birth?
- You would also be interested in ways you could help your sister manage her son's illness.

## Circuit 2/Case 9: CSA case marking sheet

### Case name: Cheryl Cameron

Case title: Common Genetic Disease
Context for the case: testing communication skills and explaining a relatively common genetic disorder

### 1. Assessment domain: Data-Gathering, Technical and Assessment Skills
Recognises concern about possible genetic disorders as the primary reason for attendance

| *Positive descriptors:* | *Negative descriptors:* |
|---|---|
| <ul><li>Takes suitable family/genetic history</li><li>Seeks information about patient's concerns for both herself and the nephew</li><li>Explores patient understanding of cystic fibrosis, including knowledge of disease, genetics and screening</li><li>Uses opportunity to enquire about pre-pregnancy issues</li></ul> | <ul><li>Fails to take adequate history about nephew and wider family</li><li>Is disorganised/unsystematic in gathering information about patient's worries and concerns</li><li>Does not explore why the patient is concerned about how the problem relates to her personally</li><li>No enquiry into patient's current feelings towards starting her own family</li></ul> |

### 2. Assessment domain: Clinical Management Skills
Manages explanations about genetics and pre-pregnancy counselling simultaneously

| *Positive descriptors:* | *Negative descriptors:* |
|---|---|
| <ul><li>Discusses cystic fibrosis in general and explains the autosomal recessive genetics and the likelihood of her own child being affected</li><li>Discusses prenatal and antenatal screening</li><li>Suggests possible resources for finding out further information, such as the Cystic Fibrosis Trust</li><li>Demonstrates knowledge of clinical genetics departments and suggests referral for screening (this will vary between areas)</li></ul> | <ul><li>Shows lack of knowledge of cystic fibrosis</li><li>Fails to discuss genetics in a broad manner</li><li>Does not offer advice about dealing with ill health in the family and what the future might hold</li><li>No follow-up arrangements and/or signposting to further information are offered</li></ul> |

### 3. Assessment domain: Interpersonal Skills
Uses good communication skills to establish rapport and motivate concordance with plan

| *Positive descriptors:* | *Negative descriptors:* |
|---|---|
| <ul><li>Shows willingness and ability to discuss a genetic problem</li><li>Explores patient's concerns in a non-judgemental manner, accepting concern for herself as well as her sister</li><li>Communicates scientific information using understandable language and checks Cheryl's understanding</li></ul> | <ul><li>Fails to respond to patient's request for further information about illness</li><li>Does not let patient guide the consultation despite obvious concern</li><li>Fails to show understanding of patient's lack of knowledge about disease and reason for wanting further information</li></ul> |

## Circuit 2/Case 10: Notes for the candidate

### In this station ...

You are a salaried GP in a surgery

### Case notes for the patient:

**Name:** Nigel Beck
**Age:** 48

### Social and family history:

Nigel is a manager at the local supermarket. He lives alone.

### Past medical history:

He rarely visits the practice but is currently being seen for an ulcer and cellulitis of his left leg.

### Current medication:

Flucloxacillin 500 mg four times daily two weeks ago; one week course
Co-amoxiclav 625 mg three times daily starting one week ago

### Last entry in records:

Last seen by the practice nurse two days ago for blood tests
Random blood glucose – 21
FBC and UE are normal

## Circuit 2/Case 10: Notes for the role-player

**Name:**   Nigel Beck
**Age:**     48 (the candidate may ask for your date of birth – please prepare one)

### Background:

- You are a 48-year-old supermarket manager.
- You have quite a good diet and try to eat plenty of fruit and veg, although you do have a thing for cake and often take home leftovers from work.
- You exercise by walking the dog, which can mean walking for a few miles.
- You don't smoke, but you do drink about half a bottle of wine per night.

### Opening statement:

'You called me in to discuss the results of my blood test from two days ago.'

### Information to give if asked by the candidate:

- You have been called in to see the doctor about the results of the blood test you had done two days ago. You have been seeing the nurse practitioner for the last couple of weeks with what was thought to be an infection in the leg, but it has not been getting any better.
- You have had two courses of antibiotics, flucloxacillin and co-amoxiclav, but, apart from making you feel a little sick, they have not made you feel any better.
- You have been a little concerned recently as you have been drinking a little more than usual and noticed that you have been getting up to pee in the night most nights. This is unusual for you, but you put it down to your age.
- The only other thing that you have noticed recently is that your eyesight has deteriorated a little and is just not as sharp as it was before.
- Otherwise you have been feeling quite well, although you have been more tired than usual recently.
- You take no medication usually and until you had this strange thing on your foot didn't really visit the doctor.
- Your brother was diagnosed with diabetes a couple of years ago, but you did not think much of it as he is very overweight and as far as you are aware overweight people are the ones who usually get diabetes.
- You are otherwise well and take no regular medication
- *Examination* – finger-prick blood glucose 21, BP 146/90, pulse 88, BMI 25. Urinalysis has shown 2+ of glucose. There are no ketones in the urine. Left leg is bandaged and the patient is not keen for you to take the dressing down as the nurse has just put it on.

### How to respond to the doctor:

- Be surprised when you are told that you are diabetic as you thought that was for fat people.
- Say that you are unsure about medication as you feel OK. Only a decent explanation and good follow-up will help you comply.
- You do not want to cut down on the amount of wine that you drink.

## Circuit 2/Case 10: CSA case marking sheet

### Case name: Nigel Beck

Case title: Type 2 Diabetes
Context for the case: assessment of a newly presenting middle-aged diabetic in primary care

### 1. Assessment domain: Data-Gathering, Technical and Assessment Skills
Recognises the presentation of Type 2 diabetes

*Positive descriptors:*
- Takes good history of symptoms that could suggest diabetes
- Rules out diabetic ketoacidosis by rechecking blood glucose and urinalysis
- Seeks information about patient risk factors for diabetes and cardiovascular disease including family history and lifestyle including diet
- Suggests appropriate examination including BP, pulse, etc.

*Negative descriptors:*
- Fails to explore the circumstances behind the patient's presentation
- Fails to seek information about diabetes and cardiovascular risk, and lifestyle factors
- Does not consider diabetic ketoacidosis
- Fails to explores social or psychological aspects of the presentation

### 2. Assessment domain: Clinical Management Skills
Manages presentation of significant hyperglycaemia in Type 2 diabetes

*Positive descriptors:*
- Makes a definite diagnosis of Type 2 diabetes
- Suggests further investigations including an HbA1c, LFTs and cholesterol (FBC and UE have already been done). An ECG would be appropriate
- Outlines medication for treating the diabetes as per NICE guidelines* and suggests starting a sulfonylurea – patient is not overweight and rapid therapeutic response required
- Educates patient about lifestyle factors that are relevant to diabetes and signposts to suitable resources such as Diabetes UK
- Discuss how this affects driving
- Arrange follow-up with either GP or nurse practitioner in the next few days to assess how the patient is getting on and recheck blood glucose levels

*Negative descriptors:*
- Is hesitant in making a diagnosis of Type 2 diabetes
- Does not discuss previous blood results and no suggestion of further investigation
- Does not offer/discuss medication as per NICE guidelines
- Lack of discussion of lifestyle factors
- Fails to arrange any follow-up for patient

* National Institute for Health and Care Excellence. *Type 2 Diabetes: the management of type 2 diabetes* (Clinical Guideline 87). London: NICE, 2009, www.nice.org.uk/guidance/cg87/resources/guidance-type-2-diabetes-pdf [accessed 15 May 2015].

continued ...

### 3. Assessment domain: Interpersonal Skills
Uses good communication skills to establish rapport and motivate concordance with plan

*Positive descriptors:*
- Good explanation of Type 2 diabetes and what it means for the patient
- Allows the patient to express his feelings towards the diagnosis
- Makes a management plan in conjunction with patient

*Negative descriptors:*
- Fails to establish a rapport with the patient and be understanding when discussing an unexpected diagnosis
- Fails to convey the severity of the diagnosis and the importance of reducing the patient's blood sugar levels
- Does little to ensure concordance with the plan by not taking patient's views into account

# Circuit 2/Case 11: Notes for the candidate

## In this station ...

You are a GP in a surgery

## Case notes for the patient:

**Name:**  Gwendolyn Smith
**Age:**    50

## Social and family history:

The patient lives with her husband Trevor, 51, who has multiple sclerosis. He has had this for many years and five years ago he gave up work. Two years ago the patient gave up work and she is now the main carer for Trevor. He has deteriorated significantly recently and has had a number of hospital admissions. It is felt that his care is now palliative and he is house bound. They have no children.

## Past medical history:

Gwendolyn suffered from anxiety many years ago.

## Current medication:

Temazepam 10 mg at night as required

## Last entry in records:

One month ago asking for more sleeping tablets. The patient appeared a little stressed at that point.

## Circuit 2/Case 11: Notes for the role-player

**Name:** Gwendolyn Smith
**Age:** 50 (the candidate may ask for your date of birth – please prepare one)

### Background:

- You are a 50-year-old female.
- You live with your husband, Trevor, who has multiple sclerosis. You are his main carer.
- You have very little extra help with him.
- You have some financial difficulties as neither of you are able to work.

### Opening statement:

'I would like to discuss my husband. His MS has worsened and he is in a lot of pain and discomfort. We feel that the end will be soon. We are scared it will be long and painful, and we would both like you to do something to make it come sooner.'

### Information to give if asked by the candidate:

- You have come in to talk about your husband, Trevor.
- Trevor is 51 and has had multiple sclerosis for a long time. He used to manage well with it and led quite an active life. However, recently the symptoms have worsened and he is now confined to a wheelchair and house bound. He has difficulties with his speech and eating, and has been in and out of hospital with various problems such as urine infections and recently pneumonia.
- No further treatment is planned for him due to the severity of the illness.
- You hate seeing your husband in pain and discomfort, and you both wish the doctor would help him to die. Your wishes are that the doctor could give him something so that he can gently slip away. You have also researched this on the internet and wish to discuss a Swiss clinic that may be able to help.
- You have very little help and are the main carer. There was some contact with the specialist nurse, but you do not feel that they have been much help.
- He has a number of medications for various things, but you are unsure of what they are.
- You are so tired and are really struggling with everything. As much as you love your husband you need a break.
- You do not sleep well and have lost your appetite. You take the occasional sleeping tablet.
- You feel your mood is low.
- Neither of you can see a good way out of this except for Trevor passing away.

### How to respond to the doctor:

- You are very upset and very tired. You are pleased just to have someone listen to you.

continued …

- You would be keen to see palliative care because even a few nights in respite would help.
- Discussion of financial help and district nurse input would also help.
- You wish to discuss the end in a non-judgemental and empathetic way.
- You accept that the doctor is not allowed to help you as long as they listen to you and offer other suggestions of things that could be done to help.
- It is so important to you to feel that someone cares and helps you.

## Circuit 2/Case 11: CSA case marking sheet

### Case name: Gwendolyn Smith

Case title: Assisted Dying
Context for the case: testing communication skills with a relative of a patient who is terminally ill

### 1. Assessment domain: Data-Gathering, Technical and Assessment Skills
Recognises the request for assisted dying

*Positive descriptors:*
- Takes in-depth social history to understand the situation the patient and husband are in
- Elicits information about the patient's own health, especially surrounding the area of depression
- Finds out about the current clinical condition of Trevor and if any follow-up is planned
- Seeks information about the patient's request for assisted dying and what she knows about it

*Negative descriptors:*
- Fails to gain an understanding of the complex situation the patient and her husband are in including the support mechanism
- Does not manage to gauge the patient's emotional and financial situation
- Does not enquire about the patient's mental health
- Fails to explore the patient's ideas behind assisted dying and her knowledge of it

### 2. Assessment domain: Clinical Management Skills
Manages patient's mental health and social situation concurrently

*Positive descriptors:*
- Discusses at length the patient and husband's social situation, and possible avenues for help including palliative care, district nurses, financial help, carers' help and respite.
- Suggests that the patient has low mood and offers management strategies for this
- Offers suggestions about ways in which the health professionals would be able to keep Trevor comfortable, but that assisted dying is illegal
- Offer suitable follow-up for the patient and her husband

*Negative descriptors:*
- Fails to address the social situation and offer referral to suitable resources
- Does not suggest that the patient may be suffering from low mood and requires help of her own
- Does not discuss the law around assisted dying
- Offers to help the patient to die
- Does not offer any suitable follow-up or safety-netting to patient

### 3. Assessment domain: Interpersonal Skills
Uses good communication skills to establish rapport and motivate concordance with plan

*Positive descriptors:*
- Shows willingness to broach difficult and sensitive issues, and shows empathy towards Gwendolyn
- Does not judge patient and accepts the very difficult situation that she is in
- Explains clearly and coherently the ethical standing around assisted suicide – assisted suicide is a criminal offence and doctors are bound by GMC guidance towards it

*Negative descriptors:*
- Fails to show sufficient respect – there is the potential here for a GP to be dismissive or very doctor-centred in his or her approach
- Fails to establish a good enough rapport with patient that allows her to feel comfortable discussing upsetting and complex issues
- Uses complex language and jargon when discussing the ethical and legal issues surrounding assisted dying

# Circuit 2/Case 12: Notes for the candidate

*In this station ...*

You are the GP in a surgery

*Case notes for the patient:*

**Name:**  Jayden Jones
**Age:**    3 months

*Social and family history:*

Jayden was born vaginally, at term with no neonatal problems. He lives with his mum, dad and brother Kai.

*Past medical history:*

None

*Current medication:*

None

*Last entry in records:*

Seen by the health visitor this morning for a routine weight.

## Circuit 2/Case 12: Notes for the role-player

**Name:**    Jayden Jones
**Age:**    3 months (the candidate may ask for son's date of birth – please prepare one)

*Background:*

- You are Alisha, 25, mother of Jayden.
- You have an older son, Kai, who is two.
- You are currently on maternity leave from your job as a beauty therapist. You have not yet decided if you will go back to work.
- You live with you partner, Jackson, who is an electrician

*Opening statement:*

'Jayden seems to be quite unsettled and is having a lot of runny poos. He also seems to have pain in his tummy.'

*Information to give if asked by the candidate:*

- Jayden was born at term by vaginal delivery.
- He was fine for the first few weeks, but recently he has been more unsettled and looks like he is in pain. You have also noticed that his stools have become a little looser and his bottom is often sore.
- Up until six weeks you were breastfeeding only, but as you also have a toddler this was becoming more unmanageable so to help you get through the day you decided to mix the breastfeeding with bottle feeds. You are keen not to go back to breastfeeding all the time.
- You saw the health visitor this morning, and he is putting on weight well, but she was concerned that he might have a cow's milk allergy and that you should ask the GP to provide you with some special milk for this.
- You are using Aptamil for Jayden as your older son was fine with it.
- Other things that you have noticed are that he can have some itchy skin and you think that the dry skin he had just after he was born is beginning to come back.
- Your older son did not have anything like this, but Jayden's dad has quite bad eczema, which can regularly flare up. He is also asthmatic.
- You are yet to try anything to help with the problems as you do not know what was causing them.
- Jayden does not seem bothered straight after food, but it seems to get worse a couple of hours later. You don't think the problem is very bad, but you would like him to be more comfortable.

*How to respond to the doctor:*

- Jayden is not here today as you did not think you would need to examine him just to give him some milk, and it is currently his nap time. You do not really see why he

continued ...

has to be seen to be given special milk as the health visitor just saw him this morning and he is quite well.
- You would struggle to afford special milk and would like it to be prescribed.
- You are surprised that you would have to give up cow's milk products as well and you think you might struggle to do this.

## Circuit 2/Case 12: CSA case marking sheet

Case title: Suspected Cow's Milk Allergy in Infancy
Context for the case: ability to assess and manage possible cow's milk protein allergy

### 1. Assessment domain: Data-Gathering, Technical and Assessment Skills
Recognises the symptoms of cow's milk allergy and its management in primary care

*Positive descriptors:*
- Seeks general information about infant – birth, feeding patterns, weight gain
- Clarifies symptoms of cow's milk allergy and likelihood of it being IgE mediated
- Elicits information about family history of atopic disease
- Clarifies management options already tried and their success
- Uses the opportunity to gain information about social circumstances

*Negative descriptors:*
- Fails to gather enough information about Jayden's symptoms
- Does not seek information about previous reactions in patient and/or take relevant family history of atopy
- Does not seek to differentiate between IgE- and non-IgE-mediated allergy

### 2. Assessment domain: Clinical Management Skills
Manages potential diagnosis of cow's milk allergy appropriately

*Positive descriptors:*
- Makes a potential diagnosis of cow's milk allergy
- Discusses what this means and what a suitable management plan would be, bearing in mind that the infant is mixed fed
- Discusses the need for mum to cut out all dairy and take supplements of calcium and vitamin D
- Offers suitable formula (can offer to look this up and do prescription later)
- Refers patient to dietician for further advice
- Explains to mother that the symptoms should improve well within the next 2–4 weeks and that you would like to see them both then, when you might suggest a home challenge with cow's milk formula to confirm diagnosis
- Suggests bringing that patient in for examination

*Negative descriptors:*
- Fails to recognise the diagnosis of non-IgE-mediated cow's milk allergy
- Does not discuss the need for mother to be on a strict milk protein-free diet and does not offer calcium and vitamin D supplements
- Does not offer correct formula (or offer to look it up) to the infant
- Does not refer to the dietician
- Does not explain to mother how long it might take for the elimination diet to work
- Does not offer follow-up in practice or even health visitor to ensure that elimination diet is working
- Does not suggest bringing Jayden in for an examination

continued …

### 3. Assessment domain: Interpersonal Skills
Uses good communication skills to establish rapport and motivate concordance with plan

*Positive descriptors:*

- Engages mother and allows her time to discuss her concerns about her son
- Explores what mother has been told about cow's milk allergy and provides further information when required
- Works in partnership, using clear and understandable language, with mother when making management plan to increase compliance

*Negative descriptors:*

- Does not listen to Alisha and allow her to explain what is happening
- Fails to assess mother's ideas on what is causing the child's symptoms and what she feels will help
- Uses a formulaic approach rather than adapting to the patient's contributions
- Limited engagement with patient and does not work with her to formulate a suitable management plan with appropriate follow-up

## Circuit 2/Case 13: Notes for the candidate

*In this station ...*

You are the GP in a surgery

*Case notes for the patient:*

**Name:** James Jardine
**Age:** 74

*Social and family history:*

James is a retired accountant. He lives with his wife.

*Past medical history:*

Hypertension – 20 years
Impaired fasting glucose test last year

*Current medication:*

Bendroflumethiazide – 2.5 mg in the morning
Atorvastatin – 40 mg at night

*Last entry in records:*

Two weeks ago when Mr Jardine had his yearly blood glucose test. HbA1c 38 mmol/L (normal range 21–41 mmol/L) and FBC and UE were normal.

## Circuit 2/Case 13: Notes for the role-player

**Name:**  James Jardine
**Age:**   74 (the candidate may ask for your date of birth – please prepare one)

### Background:

- You are a 74-year-old retired accountant.
- You do not smoke.
- You eat relatively well although you do like red meat.
- You walk your dog every day.
- You live with your wife who is also retired. She is in good health.

### Opening statement:

'I have been getting up during the night to go to the toilet and it is really beginning to annoy me as I am getting very tired.'

### Information to give if asked by the candidate:

- Recently you have had to get up during the night to pass urine, usually twice. This is really annoying and you have been feeling very tired because of it.
- You have also noticed that it takes a bit longer than before to pass urine and there can be a few dribbles at the end. When you need to go you often have to go quite quickly.
- There is no pain. You have not noticed any blood or change in colour and there is no smell to it. You might be going more than you used to during the day; you are not really sure.
- Your bowels are fine and there is no pain in your abdomen.
- You have had no erectile problems.
- You have not had any incontinence.
- You are usually well otherwise, but do take medication for your blood pressure, which has been a little high, and a tablet for your cholesterol.
- You take no herbal or over-the-counter medication.
- You take both tablets at night as you forget the one in the morning sometimes.
- A year ago you were told that you had an impaired fasting glucose and know that you are a little overweight.
- You are a little worried about prostate cancer as one of your friends died of it a couple of years back. You have put off coming to the doctor because of this.
- *Examination* (this does not need to be performed) – BP 130/88, pulse 80 regular, abdo – obese, otherwise NAD, prostate – enlarged, but firm and smooth with median sulcus felt. Genital examination – NAD. Urinalysis – neg.
- *Prompt* – say 'Do you think this is cancer?' if it is not mentioned.

### How to respond to the doctor:

- Ask if you are going to get better as you are fed up of getting out of bed during the night.
- You are keen for treatment as you want something that will work quicker than those pelvic floor exercises that women do.

## Circuit 2/Case 13: CSA case marking sheet

### Case name: James Jardine

Case title: Lower Urinary Tract Symptoms and an Enlarged Prostate
Context for the case: assessment and management of lower urinary tract symptoms (LUTS)

#### 1. Assessment domain: Data-Gathering, Technical and Assessment Skills
Recognises the symptoms of LUTS and the differential diagnosis

*Positive descriptors:*
- Obtains enough information about LUTS to give differential diagnosis
- Assesses the likelihood of serious illness causing the LUTS
- Offers appropriate examination including BP, genital, abdominal and prostate examination

*Negative descriptors:*
- Fails to seek adequate information about presentation to make diagnosis of LUTS
- Does not gather information about patient's risk factors for a serious cause of his LUTS
- Fails to offer examination, including genital and prostate
- No offer of chaperone for intimate examinations

#### 2. Assessment domain: Clinical Management Skills
Manages LUTS and likely benign prostatic hypertrophy

*Positive descriptors:*
- Makes provisional diagnosis of benign prostatic hypertrophy
- Offers blood testing for PSA. Other bloods were done two weeks ago and do not need to be repeated
- Discusses possible management options including watchful waiting and trial of medical therapy, most likely an alpha-blocker
- Organises suitable follow-up to see if medication is helping or if symptoms are worsening
- Discuss lifestyle changes that may help, especially losing weight

*Negative descriptors:*
- Fails to make a sensible diagnosis of enlarged prostate
- Does not offer PSA testing or repeats tests that were done two weeks ago
- Fails to discuss suitable management issues such as watchful waiting against medication. If prescribing medication does not discuss side effects
- Misses chance for opportunistic health promotion, especially weight loss
- No follow-up arrangements are offered

#### 3. Assessment domain: Interpersonal Skills
Uses good communication skills to establish rapport and motivate concordance with plan

*Positive descriptors:*
- Offers a comfortable environment and forms a good rapport with patient, which allows exploration of LUTS
- Explores fears regarding prostate cancer and provides some reassurance
- Explains how an enlarged prostate can reduce the urine stream and cause the symptoms that patient is experiencing in simple language
- Motivates patient to attend follow-up appointment and consider change to lifestyle factors

*Negative descriptors:*
- Fails to engage with patient, causing an uncomfortable environment to discuss urinary symptoms
- Does not allow patient the opportunity to discuss his concerns about prostate cancer
- Does not offer patient management options and allows him to choose which he finds preferable
- Lacks clarity in explaining need for follow-up to assess if medication is working and/or symptoms are worsening

# Appendix I
# RCGP Curriculum Blueprint 2015

| Theme | Curriculum capabilities/competence to be demonstrated before exit from training | GMP domain | WPBA | | | | | | | CSA | AKT |
|---|---|---|---|---|---|---|---|---|---|---|---|
| | | | CbD | COT | CEX | DOPS/CEPS | PSQ | MSF | CSR | | |
| 1: Knowing Yourself and Relating to Others | **Fitness to practise** | | | | | | | | | | |
| | Develop the attitudes and behaviours expected of a good doctor | 1, 2, 3, 4 | ✓ | ✓ | ✓ | | ✓ | ✓ | ✓ | ✓ | ✓ |
| | Manage the factors that influence your performance | 1, 2 | ✓ | | | | ✓ | ✓ | ✓ | | |
| | **Maintaining an ethical approach** | | | | | | | | | | |
| | Treat others fairly and with respect, acting without discrimination | 4 | ✓ | ✓ | ✓ | | ✓ | ✓ | ✓ | ✓ | |
| | Provide care with compassion and kindness | 4 | ✓ | ✓ | ✓ | | ✓ | ✓ | ✓ | ✓ | |
| | **Communication and consultation** | | | | | | | | | | |
| | Establish an effective partnership with patients | 3 | | ✓ | ✓ | | ✓ | ✓ | ✓ | ✓ | |
| | Maintain a continuing relationship with patients, carers and families | 3 | ✓ | ✓ | ✓ | | ✓ | ✓ | ✓ | ✓ | |
| 2: Applying Clinical Knowledge and Skill | **Data-gathering and interpretation** | | | | | | | | | | |
| | Apply a structured approach to data-gathering and investigation | 3 | ✓ | ✓ | ✓ | | | | ✓ | ✓ | ✓ |
| | Interpret findings accurately to reach a diagnosis | 2 | ✓ | ✓ | ✓ | | | | ✓ | ✓ | ✓ |
| | Demonstrate a proficient approach to clinical examination* | 1, 4 | | ✓ | | ✓ | | | ✓ | ✓ | |
| | Demonstrate a proficient approach to the performance of procedures* | 1, 4 | | ✓ | | ✓ | | | ✓ | ✓ | |

| Theme | Curriculum capabilities/competence to be demonstrated before exit from training | GMP domain | WPBA | | | | | | CSR | CSA | AKT |
|---|---|---|---|---|---|---|---|---|---|---|---|
| | | | CbD | COT | CEX | DOPS/CEPS | PSQ | MSF | | | |
| | **Making decisions** | | | | | | | | | | |
| | Adopt appropriate decision-making principles | 1, 4 | ✓ | ✓ | ✓ | | | | ✓ | ✓ | ✓ |
| | Apply a scientific and evidence-based approach | 1, 2 | ✓ | ✓ | ✓ | | | | ✓ | ✓ | ✓ |
| | **Clinical management** | | | | | | | | | | |
| | Provide general clinical care to patients of all ages and backgrounds | 1 | ✓ | ✓ | ✓ | | ✓ | ✓ | ✓ | ✓ | ✓ |
| | Adopt a structured approach to clinical management | 2 | ✓ | ✓ | ✓ | | ✓ | ✓ | ✓ | ✓ | ✓ |
| | Make appropriate use of other professionals and services | 3 | ✓ | ✓ | | | | ✓ | ✓ | ✓ | ✓ |
| | Provide urgent care when needed | 1, 2 | ✓ | | ✓ | | | ✓ | ✓ | ✓ | ✓ |
| 3: Managing Complex and Long-Term Care | **Managing medical complexity** | | | | | | | | | | |
| | Enable people living with long-term conditions to improve their health | 4 | ✓ | ✓ | ✓ | | ✓ | ✓ | ✓ | ✓ | ✓ |
| | Manage concurrent health problems in an individual patient | 1 | ✓ | ✓ | ✓ | | | | ✓ | ✓ | ✓ |
| | Adopt safe and effective approaches for patients with complex health needs | 2 | ✓ | ✓ | ✓ | | ✓ | | ✓ | ✓ | |
| | **Working with colleagues and in teams** | | | | | | | | | | |
| | Work as an effective team member | 3 | ✓ | | ✓ | | ✓ | ✓ | ✓ | ✓ | |
| | Coordinate a team-based approach to the care of patients | 3 | ✓ | ✓ | ✓ | | | ✓ | ✓ | ✓ | |

| Theme | Curriculum capabilities/competence to be demonstrated before exit from training | GMP domain | WPBA | | | | | | | | AKT |
|---|---|---|---|---|---|---|---|---|---|---|---|
| | | | CbD | COT | CEX | DOPS/CEPS | PSQ | MSF | CSR | CSA | |
| | **Maintaining performance, learning and teaching** | | | | | | | | | | |
| 4: Working Well in Organisations and Systems of Care | Continuously evaluate and improve the care you provide | 2, 4 | ✓ | | | | ✓ | ✓ | ✓ | | |
| | Adopt a safe and scientific approach to improve quality of care | 2 | ✓ | | | | | | ✓ | | ✓ |
| | Support the education and development of colleagues | 3 | ✓ | | | | ✓ | ✓ | ✓ | | |
| | **Organisational management and leadership** | | | | | | | | | | |
| | Apply leadership skills to help improve your organisation's performance | 1 | ✓ | | | | | | ✓ | | |
| | Develop the financial and business skills required for your role | 4 | ✓ | | | | | ✓ | ✓ | | ✓ |
| | Make effective use of information management and communication systems | 3 | ✓ | ✓ | ✓ | | ✓ | ✓ | ✓ | ✓ | ✓ |
| 5: Caring for the Whole Person and the Wider Community | **Practising holistically and promoting health** | | | | | | | | | | |
| | Demonstrate the holistic mindset of a generalist medical practitioner | 1 | ✓ | ✓ | | | ✓ | ✓ | ✓ | ✓ | |
| | Support people through individual experiences of health, illness and recovery | 4 | ✓ | ✓ | | | ✓ | ✓ | ✓ | ✓ | |
| | **Community orientation** | | | | | | | | | | |
| | Understand the health service and your role within it | 2 | ✓ | ✓ | | | | | ✓ | ✓ | ✓ |
| | Build relationships with the communities with which you work | 3 | ✓ | | | | ✓ | ✓ | ✓ | | |

* These new *Clinical examination and procedural skills* competences have been introduced to replace DOPS.

*Note:* The general practice curriculum is divided into six areas of competence and three 'essential features', which are described in detail in the first of the curriculum statements, *Being a General Practitioner*. The assessment blueprint shows how these areas of competence and essential features relate to the four domains of *Good Medical Practice* (1: Knowledge, skills and performance, 2: Safety and quality, 3: Communication, partnership and teamwork, and 4: Maintaining trust).

The curriculum statements produced by the Royal College of General Practitioners are as follows:

**1: Being a General Practitioner**

**2: The Contextual Statements**

2.01 The GP Consultation in Practice

2.02 Patient Safety and Quality of Care

2.03 The GP in the Wider Professional Environment

2.04 Enhancing Professional Knowledge

**3: The Clinical Examples**

3.01 Healthy People: Promoting Health and Preventing Disease

3.02 Genetics in Primary Care

3.03 Care of Acutely Ill People

3.04 Care of Children and Young People

3.05 Care of Older Adults

3.06 Women's Health

3.07 Men's Health

3.08 Sexual Health

3.09 End-of-Life Care

3.10 Care of People with Mental Health Problems

3.11 Care of People with Intellectual Disability

3.12 Cardiovascular Health

3.13 Digestive Health

3.14 Care of People who Misuse Drugs and Alcohol

The blueprint also indicates how each of these domains and essential features are tested across the three components of the GP licensing examination, namely WPBA, CSA and AKT.

The areas of competence and essential features are generic elements of performance, and the manner in which each of these generic areas are applied to specified contexts is described in the curriculum statements, which are listed below.

3.15 Care of People with ENT, Oral and Facial Problems

3.16 Care of People with Eye Problems

3.17 Care of People with Metabolic Problems

3.18 Care of People with Neurological Problems

3.19 Respiratory Health

3.20 Care of People with Musculoskeletal Problems

3.21 Care of People with Skin Problems

*Glossary*

AKT: Applied Knowledge Test (computer-marked multiple-choice paper)

CbD: Case-based Discussion

CEPS: Clinical Examination and Procedural Skills

CEX: Clinical Evaluation Exercise

COT: Consultation Observation Tool

CSA: Clinical Skills Assessment (OSCE-type examination)

CSR: clinical supervisor's report

DOPS: Direct Observation of Procedural Skills

GMP: *Good Medical Practice*

MSF: Multi-Source Feedback

PSQ: Patient Satisfaction Questionnaire

WPBA: Workplace-Based Assessment

# Appendix II
# Generic marking indicators for the three marking domains in the CSA

## 1. DATA-GATHERING, TECHNICAL AND ASSESSMENT SKILLS
Gathering and using data for clinical judgement, choice of examination, investigations and their interpretation. Demonstrating proficiency in performing physical examinations and using diagnostic and therapeutic instruments (*blueprint: Problem-Solving Skills, Technical Skills*).

*Positive indicators*
- Clarifies the problem and nature of decision required
- Uses an incremental approach, using time and accepting uncertainty
- Gathers information from history taking, examination and investigation in a systematic and efficient manner
- Is appropriately selective in the choice of enquiries, examinations and investigations
- Identifies abnormal findings or results and makes appropriate interpretations
- Uses instruments appropriately and fluently
- When using instruments or conducting physical examinations, performs actions in a rational sequence

*Negative indicators*
- Makes immediate assumptions about the problem
- Intervenes rather than using appropriate expectant management
- Is disorganised/unsystematic in gathering information
- Data-gathering does not appear to be guided by the probabilities of disease
- Fails to identify abnormal data or correctly interpret them
- Appears unsure of how to operate/use instruments
- Appears disorganised/unsystematic in the application of the instruments or the conduct of physical examinations

## 2. CLINICAL MANAGEMENT SKILLS
Recognition and management of common medical conditions in primary care. Demonstrating a structured and flexible approach to decision-making. Demonstrating the ability to deal with multiple complaints and co-morbidity. Demonstrating the ability to promote a positive approach to health (*blueprint: Primary Care Management, Comprehensive Approach*).

*Positive indicators*
- Recognises presentations of common physical, psychological and social problems
- Makes plans that reflect the natural history of common problems
- Offers appropriate and feasible management options
- Management approaches reflect an appropriate assessment of risk
- Makes appropriate prescribing decisions
- Refers appropriately and coordinates care with other healthcare professionals

*Negative indicators*
- Fails to consider common conditions in the differential diagnosis
- Does not suggest how the problem might develop or resolve
- Fails to make the patient aware of relative risks of different approaches
- Decisions on whether/what to prescribe are inappropriate or idiosyncratic
- Decisions on whether and where to refer are inappropriate.
- Follow-up arrangements are absent or disjointed

- Manages risk effectively, safety-netting appropriately
- Simultaneously manages multiple health problems, both acute and chronic
- Encourages improvement, rehabilitation, and, where appropriate, recovery
- Encourages the patient to participate in appropriate health promotion and disease prevention strategies

- Fails to take account of related issues or of co-morbidity
- Unable to construct a problem list and prioritise
- Unable to enhance patient's health perceptions and coping strategies

## 3. INTERPERSONAL SKILLS

Demonstrating the use of recognised communication techniques to gain understanding of the patient's illness experience and develop a shared approach to managing problems. Practising ethically with respect for equality and diversity issues, in line with the accepted codes of professional conduct (*blueprint: Person-Centred Approach, Attitudinal Aspects*).

*Positive indicators*

- Explores patient's agenda, health beliefs and preferences
- Appears alert to verbal and non-verbal cues
- Explores the impact of the illness on the patient's life
- Elicits psychological and social information to place the patient's problem in context
- Works in partnership, finding common ground to develop a shared management plan
- Communicates risk effectively to patients
- Shows responsiveness to the patient's preferences, feelings and expectations
- Enhances patient autonomy
- Provides explanations that are relevant and understandable to the patient
- Responds to needs and concerns with interest and understanding
- Has a positive attitude when dealing with problems, admits mistakes and shows commitment to improvement
- Backs own judgement appropriately
- Demonstrates respect for others
- Does not allow own views/values to influence dialogue inappropriately
- Shows commitment to equality of care for all
- Acts in an open, non-judgemental manner
- Is cooperative and inclusive in approach
- Conducts examinations with sensitivity for the patient's feelings, seeking consent where appropriate

*Negative indicators*

- Does not enquire sufficiently about the patient's perspective/health understanding
- Pays insufficient attention to the patient's verbal and non-verbal communication
- Fails to explore how the patient's life is affected by the problem
- Does not appreciate the impact of the patient's psychosocial context
- Instructs the patient rather than seeking common ground
- Uses a rigid approach to consulting that fails to be sufficiently responsive to the patient's contribution
- Fails to empower the patient or encourage self-sufficiency
- Uses inappropriate (e.g. technical) language
- Shows little visible interest/understanding, lacks warmth in voice/manner
- Avoids taking responsibility for errors
- Does not show sufficient respect for others
- Inappropriately influences patient interaction through own views/values
- Treats issues as problems rather than challenges
- Displays inappropriate favour or prejudice
- Is quick to judge
- Appears patronising or inappropriately paternalistic
- When conducting examinations, appears unprofessional and at risk of hurting or embarrassing the patient

*Source:* www.rcgp.org.uk/gp-training-and-exams/mrcgp-exams-overview/~/media/
BD43B1D830F14793A92C505360F50D08.ashx.

# Appendix III
# Hospital letter

Royal Hospital
Addiscombe Lane
London

Dear Doctor,

**Re: Mark Horner (son of the late Mr John Horner)**

Mr John Horner (aged 65) died of liver failure in this unit one year ago. The underlying cause was discovered to be haemochromatosis. As you know this is an autosomal recessive genetic condition.

We have written to Mr Mark Horner advising him that his father died of a genetic disorder and have advised him to consult you regarding future investigations.

Thank you for your help in this matter.

Yours faithfully,

Dr Toby Smith
Dept of Gastroenterology

# Appendix IV
# Complex case – Mr J

```
1  CAN:  hello hi there come in
2  RPL:  hi doctor hi thank you
3  CAN:  mr j*****
4  RPL:  yeah that's right yes
5        (pause)
6  CAN:  my name is dr xxxxx how can I help you this morning
7  RPL:  um I'd like a referral for a vasectomy please
8  CAN:  right (.) ok um you must have been thinking about that for **** **** ok
9  RPL:  yeah I suppose so yes yes yes
10 CAN:  tell me a little bit about your thoughts about it
11 RPL:  um well I know that I've I've (.) never wanted children
12 CAN:  right
13 RPL:  and I know that I
14 RPL:  never do
15 CAN:  ok
16 RPL:  so um you know it feels like the the more rational permanent choice really
17 CAN:  ok um tell me a little bit about what you know about vasectomy already
18 RPL:  um
19 CAN:  have you done any reading or have you spoken to anybody about it
20 RPL:  yeah I've spoken to a few people at k- er a few of the guys at work have had it
21        have had it successfully done
22        um I suppose my knowledge is fairly general I know it's (.) a fairly brief
23 CAN:  yep
24 RPL:  procedure um and can be
25 CAN:  it is yes
26 RPL:  you know back to work the next day
27 CAN:  ok
28 RPL:  yep
29 CAN:  ok so it sounds like you know a little bit
30 RPL:  a little bit yeah
31 CAN:  maybe I could give you a few more details
32 RPL:  mmm yeah yeah
33 CAN:  um there's a very (.) well it's a very effective procedure but it's something
34        with quite permanent consequences
35 RPL:  mmm mmm
36 CAN:  which is something that we will go over um I haven't met you before
37 RPL:  no
38 CAN:  I do have a few details in your records I notice that you're not currently in a relationship
```

```
39 RPL:   oh I am yes yes yes yes
40 CAN:   oh you are ok can you tell me a bit about that
41 RPL:   oh well I mean we've been together for a long time I mean yeah I mean I I
42 CAN:   mmhmm
43 RPL:   seldom need to come in here so I don't know how old the records are but er
44 CAN:   oh they must be quite old
45 RPL:   er b- yeah I mean we've we've lived together for years so
46 CAN:   right
47 RPL:   yeah
48 CAN:   ok and is this um is this a decision that you've taken together is it something that
49 RPL:   um I'd probably say it's my decision
50 CAN:   ok
51 RPL:   ummm last time we chatted about things was a few years ago
52 CAN:   ok
53 RPL:   and I know that we didn't want any children then and I know that
54 CAN:   yeah yes
55 RPL:   I don't want any children now so so I feel as though you know
56 CAN:   yeah
57 RPL:   it's my decision to make
58 CAN:   ok is your partner female male
59 RPL:   yes female yeah
60 CAN:   if you mind me asking ok and is there something now er er I know you've just said it's your
61        decision to make
62 RPL:   mmm
63 CAN:   and I completely agree
64 RPL:   mmm
65 CAN:   is it something that she's aware that you've been thinking about is it something that you've
66        talked about (.) together
67 RPL:   er no
68 CAN:   right
69 RPL:   no I mean it's you know I I I feel as though I'd I'd (.) prefer to do it to do it myself er
70 CAN:   ok
71 RPL:   yeah
72 CAN:   do you mind me asking for what reason
73 RPL:   um I I have a slight inkling that she might be a bit little bit broody at the moment
74 CAN:   right
75 RPL:   um and um I know that I (.) don't want to make her pregnant
76 CAN:   ok
77 RPL:   um (.) so I feel as though (.) this is
78 RPL:   my choice to make I suppose
79 CAN:   ok
80 RPL:   yeah
81 CAN:   have you considered any other options that might be available to you
82 RPL:   er as far as I can tell the other options seem to be from for (.) her
83 CAN:   yes
84 RPL:   as opposed to for me and and and as this feels as though it's a decision which I'd like to make
85        myself and um
86 CAN:   right
87 RPL:   then there are few options
88 CAN:   ok yeah
89 RPL:   than I suppose
90 CAN:   I can see the difficulties that lie there
```

```
■1        right it's a slightly unusual request I mean I see people quite often asking for a vasectomies
■2        they tend to be men who are a little bit older who already have a family
■3 RPL:   mmm
 4 CAN:   um so it's unusual in in that respect
■5 RPL:   mmm
■6 CAN:   the other thing is that without your partner knowing I mean this is in most cases a permanent
■7        (.) operation
■8 RPL:   mmm
■9 CAN:   which again I said we'll go into in just a minute
.00       so it's maybe some things to think about there and we'll go through that together
.01 RPL:  mmm
.02 CAN:  ok um do you want me to give you a few more details on vasectomy just as as we're discussing
03        this (.) ok
.04 RPL:  yep yep mmm
05 CAN:   well like you said….
```

# Index